Our Biology Runs Deep

Our Biology Runs Deep

Consciousness Building from Multiple Perspectives

Roger A. Williamson, MD

HYPERBARIC PRESS ⁘ IOWA CITY

Hyperbaric Press, Iowa City, Iowa, 52240
Copyright © 2022 Roger A. Williamson, MD
Published in association with Catstep Press, Iowa City, Iowa
ISBN: 978-0-9828477-3-2

To my siblings, Tim, left, and Marilyn

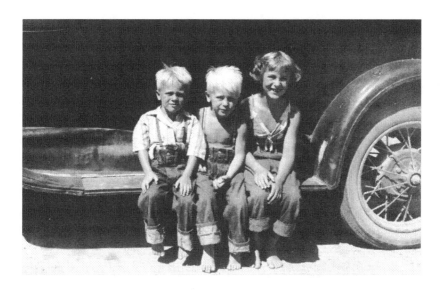

Contents

Preface

WHAT BEGAN AS AN effort to understand and write about the theories of consciousness from a basic science perspective has become an amalgam. We intuitively know consciousness on a superficial plane, our awareness of our internal and external existence, but on a deeper level questions abound. My initial forays into this enigmatic field were severely wanting. I began to reason the only way I might be able to meaningfully contribute to this topic would be via a personal history, followed by selected areas of science informed by these reflections. It, therefore, became a goal to use autobiography in the service of narrowing the scientific focus. Personal details of a life would not flow seamlessly into an examination of consciousness, but I believed I could merge the separate streams to achieve a credible level of complementarity.

As I was writing a personal narrative, I realized that calibrating the amount of detail was a balance that is not easily negotiated. I initially included a series of remembrances which would interest my siblings. This reminiscing inevitably expanded to become not only a tribute to them, but also to peers, colleagues, and mentors I have admired. What we bring to a project such as this is a rich combination of the propensities we are born with and the environments we live within, most tellingly our families, schools, and workplaces. I have trusted that this level of detail will not detract from the overriding theme, consciousness.

Among evolved human traits, none has produced the wonder accorded the attainment of consciousness. Our human abilities to reason, pursue the arts, express a range of emotions and interpret and react to complex emotions of others, consider the past, and conjecture about the future has evolved over the vastness of time. From the earliest history of life our ancestors, from bacteria onward, have had "awareness" of the environment, the ability to attend to their surroundings, and possessed the competitive armamentarium to assure survival. The sensing systems which organisms employ are engineering marvels. Understanding how the senses transmit information from the external world to the interior continues to be an active area of research in all life forms and contributes to a fuller picture of human sentience.

But understanding how the human brain bundles sensory information—sights, sounds, smells, taste, and touch—co-mingled with thoughts, memories, and emotions to produce an ongoing, coherent stream of consciousness is a huge chasm. We may not bridge this chasm. It remains an open question whether science can reveal the slow, arduous steps whereby this special attribute became manifest. Many fine minds, however, have not been deterred. A compulsion born of intense curiosity compels scholars to ponder big questions. It was inevitable that this intriguing topic, consciousness, became a scientific quarry.

Consciousness came to its present state of expression in humans through myriad, small genetic changes over billions of years of collective inheritance. These variations have influenced structure and behavior, broadly defined as the response of an organism to varying conditions imposed by a mutually interacting and reinforcing environment. This is a highly competitive process. Consciousness emerged as successive combinatorial possibilities of elements, be they particles of the quantum world, atoms, molecules, or cells, produced structural and functional modifications that survived the natural selection process, thereby serving as substrates for further change. The concept of emergence is edifying in the context of the vastness of the possible arrangements of the building blocks of consciousness. Emergence is the concept that when constituent elements combine to produce higher-order, functional properties, the result of that combination is more complex than the sum of the starting elements.[1]

Highly personal details of a life, painful as they are to relate, prompt reflection and can be a source of intuition and insight into a deeper understanding of reality, and hence consciousness. In this work I will endeavor to relate psychological insights to the consuming puzzle of consciousness. I will trace some of the deep roots of the biological basis of emotions and will posit that aspects of emotion, particularly its dysregulation, could plausibly have contributed to the development of consciousness.

CHAPTER 1

A Personal Narrative

I ARRIVED AS QUICKLY AS FEASIBLE after receiving the call that my father was gravely ill. The nurse pointed me to a room with the identifying tag, Tom Williamson. As I eased into his hospital room, I became painfully aware of the reason I was awakened early that morning. On first view, his abdomen was grotesquely swollen, elevating the bed sheets above the railing, this smooth mound towering above his sunken chest. The head of the bed was elevated. When his eyes opened, he offered a brief nod. I was unprepared for his gaunt expression. I was as unprepared for this encounter as any son would be, made more poignant by a fraught relationship extending as far back as meaningful memory. To this day I wonder why it was my number he offered as emergency contact.

He had entered the hospital in Pueblo, Colorado for what was scheduled to be a "routine" gall bladder removal after months of vague abdominal pain. His cirrhotic liver could not have been missed had proper screening been done. It is probable this scarred organ was so compromised it could not metabolize the anesthetics. This led, inevitably, to liver failure and the accumulation of fluid in his abdomen. In medical school I had learned in excruciating detail the pathophysiology leading to the state my father was in, memorizing the causes of cirrhosis and tipping points wherein one or a few more insults begin the deadly cascade of events.

The operating surgeon's partner, the person who had made the initial phone call, did not speculate about a cause, and had called in consultants. Dad was frightened and a little confused. However, he was able to recall that in San Francisco, during a period when I would have been a young child, he had become jaundiced, suggesting liver disease. This was likely the inciting event. Further hospital tests implicated one of the viruses which can infect the liver, hepatitis B, transmitted by bodily fluids, often sexually. Given his history, this is the most likely mode of transmission, though it remains a possibility that dad contracted the disease via a finger stick by an infected needle. Some who become infected with hepatitis B develop chronic active hepatitis, which can result in end-stage liver failure after a struggle between the destructive bent of the virus and the reparative mechanisms of the liver. The virus had been a hidden, stalking alien, inexorably destroying his liver over many decades, cell by cell.

Bill, dad's current partner with whom he was living in Rye, 35 miles south of Pueblo, spent most of his time in the waiting room. When in dad's room he remained on the periphery, looking puzzled but asking no questions, having little conception of this sudden transformation. He frequently retreated to the safety of the smoking zone outdoors. Bill was raised in the hills of Tennessee. He was younger than dad, unschooled in the arts or literature; it was an incongruous match when viewed from a distance. As I came to appreciate in later years, dad had consuming emotional needs and Bill met enough of them. I surmise dad could not risk another partner comparable to him in intellect and aesthetic leanings whose departure could precipitate descent into a depressive Hell.

I called my unsuspecting siblings, sister Marilyn, and brother Tim. I remained with him for several days. We talked sparingly and superficially. This was not the setting to dredge the past, put a different interpretation on it, try a new understanding. The end was near; this realization superseded all others. When I again called Tim to tell him I needed to return to my work as a relatively new faculty member of the department of Ob/Gyn at the medical school in Iowa City, Iowa, he flew to Colorado from his residence in California and was at dad's side when he expired. Dad was given to singing. Tim relates that in a moment of lucidity before dying he sang, *I'm Forever Blowing Bubbles.*

After church service in Rye, a small band of people filed through the rain, umbrellas splayed, to his gravesite at the back of the cemetery. Mother had come to the funeral from her home in Rifle, the home my sibs and I mostly grew up in, a small town on the western slope of Colorado. As we walked back from the burial and she was preparing to leave, mother told me, in her quiet, reserved manner, that a physician had recently felt a mass in her lower abdomen and was going to operate. By her description I was concerned it may be ovarian cancer. My training informed me that the optimal chance to cure or prolong life of those with this dreaded disease involved extensive surgery, with dissection and removal of long chains of lymph nodes, a procedure beyond the capabilities of an Ob/Gyn physician who did not have additional years of training.

Before her proposed surgery I went back to Rifle and requested a meeting with her physician. I indicated he and I had the same training, and I certainly did not feel capable of performing an adequate surgery for this disease, assuming it was ovarian cancer. He was not deterred. My brother, a pediatrician, and I knew surgeons at other institutions capable of optimal removal of this tumor, often widespread throughout the abdomen by the time it was symptomatic and detected.

Mother felt more comfortable staying near home; we honored her wish. She, unfortunately, had ovarian cancer and the surgery was inadequate. She subsequently agreed to go to UCLA, near Tim's home in Ojai, California, where a more complete surgery was performed. Following surgery, she endured multiple courses of grueling, debilitating chemotherapy. Marilyn, now a high school teacher in Rifle and always close to mother, ever helpful and caring, was on the front line. During one hospitalization for another round of chemotherapy in Grand Junction, 60 miles down the highway from Rifle, mother's white blood cell count—cells on which she depended to ward off infection—dropped to a dangerously low level. She became overwhelmingly infected (septic) and rapidly died. We gathered in Rifle to bury the woman who had sacrificed so much for her children. Both parents were just 63.

Everyone has a story. All are complicated, many are interesting, and some are instructive. Parents are central to many of these narratives. Mine were disparate in many fundamental aspects. Mother was reserved, responsible, and, at times of her life, cripplingly anxious. Marilyn and Tim would probably describe her as selfless; I have tended to regard her as dutiful, though the margins are blurred. My siblings shared more with her than I allowed and would regard her as warm and nurturing. I did not sense these attributes to the degree they did but would never describe her as cold or withdrawn. She thought deeply about politics and took well-reasoned positions on topics like finance and the economy. Her view of the world was a conservative one. Her brother said that as a child she was lively. When they visited relatives in eastern Colorado as children, she rode horses with the best of them and was a good shot with a rifle when rabbit hunting. From my earliest memories of her onward, she seemed to have lost this spunk.

Dad, by contrast, could command attention, be showy, was an avowed romantic, was occasionally impulsive, and certainly subject to the vagaries of mood. He was also creative. He was a self-taught artist. I would judge his oil paintings to have been passable to quite good. He favored wildlife, particularly birds, though his signature pieces were clowns, the sadness leeching from their garish, paint-smeared expressions and entreating stares. He painted a pretty, teenage boy with blond hair and reddish lips, a painting I still have, along with some others. He held one-person shows and sold much of his art. His emotional life was never far below the painted surface. He was self-absorbed in his strivings for connectedness and love. These strivings were sometimes thwarted. When this happened, he became dangerously depressed. But most of this remained hidden to me. With all his activities, viewed from afar, he seemed the elusive, interesting one. He was the absent figure, pursuing an exotic life. Growing up I craved his withheld affection and attention.

How did we get to this juncture, the deaths of parents, one who, over time, engendered deep ambivalence, and the other, the caretaker whose life was one of denial, always submerging her interests? For his part, dad left a written family history which has helped me understand him to a degree. He was the middle of three brothers, born to a hard charging, general practitioner father, Arthur, and a headstrong, artistic mother, Georgeanne. They lived in Pueblo, variously known at that time as Steel City or as the Pittsburgh of the West. Foreign laborers were needed for the smelters, coal mines, and other strenuous jobs. A large proportion of these jobs were filled by immigrants from Sicily and Italy, fleeing economic hard times. Others of this immigrant population eschewed these demanding jobs, turning to bootlegging in the era of prohibition and other money generating enterprises. Prior to 1920 the "Mafia" was known as the "Black Hand," their activities in Colorado extending from the New Mexico border north to Denver. In Pueblo members were known as "The Sicilian Organization." There were rival factions and murders were common. [1]

Dad's father practiced medicine and surgery during this era. By dad's description, he was an ebullient, colorful character. He chose a solo practice rather than joining one of the two established groups in Pueblo. His large clientele included a significant proportion of Sicilian and Italian families. Dad was in awe of his father, often accompanying him on house calls. He relates the demonstrative shows of affection when his father would enter the house of one of these immigrant families. The language of these first-generation immigrants was a limiting factor, but sheer emotion and gestures likely allowed the rudiments of communication. His father was as voluble and mercurial as his patients. Most of these immigrants who were his patients were not involved in illegal activities, but some were. There was a tacit understanding; he would not ask about their livelihoods, and they would never ask for favors such as "a doctor's excuse" for their whereabouts following a nefarious deed. Did he compromise his morality? His code allowed for this behavior, and the pact he had with these families doubtless served emotional needs on both sides. He attended many of their celebrations and had delivered many of their children, sometimes using what was known locally as "Dr. Williamson's spoon," no doubt one of the early forceps then available. When he died at age 50 from sepsis, secondary to a middle ear infection, his wife said no one was to be turned away from the service. The church overflowed with mourners, many of whom were Italian women, draped in black shawls, and their families. An entire wall was blanketed with red roses and an overhead sign in gold letters proclaiming, "The Sicilian Organization."

Dad declared his love for his father in writing. When his father died, he was only 14. The loss deeply saddened him and was likely to impact his reaction to future losses. His childhood prior to this death was, by his telling, a happy one. The summers were spent in the small town of Rye, within the San Isabel National Forest and abutting the Greenhorn Range, a town to which he retreated on numerous occasions, the town he chose to live out his last days. His dad had built a small log cabin in 1927 on a plot of land sufficient to raise a horse or two.

Horses were a fixture in dad's life until his death, with a decided preference for the Arabian breed. Once, while riding his horse near Rye as a youngster, a couple sitting on their porch waved and he rode over to pay respects. This couple, Marie and Raymond Bell, were kind, generous people who became a part of the family. They helped dad at many junctures with their sensitive listening. Years ago, I went back to Rye to find dad's grave. Toward the back of the cemetery I found his small headstone atop an unkempt plot. Close by Marie and Raymond were buried. There was also a tiny headstone for their infant, born with severe birth defects. Dad indicated Marie had other pregnancies resulting in miscarriages, but no living children.

Georgeanne was now his major influence. She expected that after high school he would major in pre-med. His older brother had become a doctor, and it was apparently his mother's expectation he would also follow this path. Dad initially balked, enrolling in college to become a forest ranger. After two years he complied with his mother's wishes, finished his pre-medical studies and was accepted to the medical school in Denver, enrolling in 1938. His emotional vulnerabilities were quickly and starkly unmasked. He deeply disliked the subject matter, sights, and odors. These all folded into his confusion and were a harbinger of later tumult. He did poorly, and after a quarter dropped out. In his family history he relates he "flunked out." Following more undergraduate work he was allowed to re-enroll, but after buying his books and a microscope, he realized he would again be unable to do the work; hence more confusion, emotional discord, and scrambling to find a life's work, knowing he was disappointing his mother.

He decided to become a teacher and enrolled at Western State College in Gunnison to pursue that goal. There he met my mother, Helen Yates, then secretary to the president of the college. They married in 1940. There was little information in his family history about their courtship. He was offered a position teaching science at Rye High School where he joined six other teachers. He left after a year, ostensibly because the salary was so low. He and mother moved into the basement of her father's home in Denver, a refuge on multiple occasions for members of the family following some dislocation or other.

After several other marginal jobs and a child (Marilyn, born in 1941), he took the decision to re-apply to medical school and was again accepted. It would be interesting to know his deliberations and those of the selection committee. Why would the committee take a chance on him again, and why would he subject himself to a profession he seemed so uncomfortable with? It no doubt helped that he was inducted into the army, which paid for his schooling.

He persevered and made it through. I was born in 1944, a year before his graduation. He was accepted into an internship in Portland where Tim was born, 15 months following my birth. We were back in grandfather's house in Denver after internship while dad was sent to Officer's Training School in Texas, where he received orders to report for two years of duty in the Army Medical Corps at Ft. Lewis, Washington. We left Denver and joined him.

After his service obligations, we were back in grandfather's basement as a family. It was at this time dad drove with a friend to the western slope of Colorado to find a suitable place to start a practice. When they stopped for gas, dad spotted a sign, "O. F. Clagett, MD." He knocked, and an older, white-haired gentleman answered the door. Dr. Clagett had contracted tuberculosis in Missouri, and was advised to move to a higher altitude, a move which proved to be salutary. The two of them talked a short while. Dr. Clagett, a revered practitioner, seemed to signal dad would be welcome in this ranching and farming community of about 2,000 residents. An impulsive but fortuitous decision was made on the spot, fortuitous because dad, unsure of his abilities, would have a highly competent physician he could call upon for help and advice. Dad did not suddenly shed his intimidation of the responsibilities of caring for sick patients. He still harbored the fear of and disdain for medicine that drove him from medical school on his first attempt.

If he was aided in so many ways by Dr. Clagett, and he surely was, real help was on the way. The Rye couple, Marie and Raymond Bell, had recently lost their child with multiple birth defects and they were grieving. Dad offered solace and a plea; come to Rifle where Raymond could help build a house and Marie, with no prior experience, could be "trained" by dad to be his office nurse. They were a stabilizing influence. Once dad was able to pasture a horse close by, this also had a beneficial effect.

Until I began a to do little digging, I had forgotten that Dr. Clagett had a son, O. T. (Jim) Clagett, who went through the Rifle school system years ahead of me. He also became a physician, one well-regarded in academic circles. He co-founded the department of cardiovascular surgery at Mayo Clinic in Rochester, Minnesota. He had been president of the American Association of Thoracic Surgery, among other honors. Each year at Mayo the division of general thoracic surgery hosts the O. T. Clagett Visiting Professor. When I was in medical school making rounds with the thoracic surgery team, I recall a patient whose lung had been removed and the space the lung previously occupied had become infected, filled with pus. The space had been drained, and the discussion that morning turned to instillation of an antibiotic solution to cause the linings of the space to fuse, thus obliterating the cavity to prevent further infection. I was unaware at the time that this two-stage procedure is called the Clagett procedure.[2,3] In an ironic, cruel happenstance of fate, another of Dr. Clagett's accomplished sons fell to his death while climbing the Flatirons on the edge of Boulder, Colorado, near the house dad lived in for many years.

Had it not been for the encouragement and backing of Dr. Clagett and the subsequent presence of the Bells, I doubt dad would have been able to practice for over two years in Rifle. Though he shared some coverage with the osteopathic physician in town, his freedom was obviously constrained. Even after his practice was well established, his discomfort with sickness and emergencies had never fully abated since similar feelings had put him to flight the first time he enrolled in medical school. And always, in the background, was his submerged sexuality. In the era he practiced medicine, homosexuality was widely thought to be deviant. This orientation was officially considered an illness by the medical establishment and was so codified in the extant version of the Diagnostic and Statistical Manual of the American Psychiatric Association. Treatments here and abroad were ineffective, and some were dangerous. It is harrowing to read the story of Alan Turing, the Brit who cracked the Enigma code in WWII. He submitted to hormone treatments rather than going to jail for the "crime" of homo-sexuality and later committed suicide.[4]

I can only surmise that the relatively rough-hewn population of Rifle, or almost any place in America at that time, would recoil in revulsion to know their physician was gay. Dad remained tightly, deeply closeted. His seques-tered urges were never in evidence. He had no "mannerisms" or patterns of speech which would betray his sexuality. He had, after all, produced a three-child façade. The toll on him had to have been immense. One might assume he was bisexual; he was not. The only time the topic was discussed between us, maybe five years from his death, he indicated he had known since age 12 that his sexual interests were exclusively for males. In his family history there was no mention of the subject, but he placed several poems he had written at the end of the history, one a paean to San Francisco and a lover he titled *San Francisco—City of Mystery*. The concluding stanza reads:

Goodnight, My Darling, in dreams you'll be near,
I would you were close that you might hear,
My lips repeat what my heart sang all day,
I love you, My Darling, near, or away.

Earlier stanzas in this verse betray his lover is a man. The prose is sophomoric. It was written in 1949, when I was five. He was obviously traveling to San Francisco at various times. Was the addition of this poem to his written history his way to confess, to tell anyone reading the history that he was gay, that he had accepted it and so should the reader? Was the object of his affection the person from whom he contracted hepatitis B? Or was the viral infection the result of a quick, frenzied coupling with someone anonymous and faceless?

Was mother aware? I can't imagine she wasn't. Tim knew they were not sleeping together, a fact he shared much later in life. Though the following story may be apocryphal, I seem to recall that as children Tim and I were driven by mother to Denver to have our "hormones checked." Mother would certainly want to know if either of us was predisposed, and to do anything possible to steer a different course. If this scenario is true, faulty science was at the base. And if true, the assessment must have been OK; I don't recall a follow-up.

In the first and second grades it became evident to me that all was not well in my parents' relationship. I recall one tense exchange in the kitchen when I was assumed to be asleep on the couch. Dad was insistently pressing his points; she was standing her ground. A memory was seared. I am sure there were many other heated arguments from which we were shielded. I was becoming sensitive to strife, discord, and tension, and developing a life-long aversion to conflict of any stripe.

I was also becoming acutely sensitive to personal foibles and perceived failures. In our second-grade play, *Peter Cottontail*, I joined the others donning a bunny outfit. At a dramatic point in the production, I was to heave a carrot across the stage. I had rehearsed the scene many times. But no, the carrot was launched early, much to my embarrassment; another seared memory. At the start of the first or second grade I recall another scene with a youngster's version of great empathy. We were, individually by row, to stand before our seated classmates and state our name and what we did over the summer. There were few truly poor people in Rifle, but one shabbily dressed girl stood speechless while urine dribbled down her leg and pooled at her feet. From time to time, I reflect on that scene. Despite all the talks and lectures I have given, I never overcame the discomfort of being in front of a crowd.

In the early months of my second grade, dad moved to San Francisco. His absence remained unexplained, and I did not inquire. The following summer the family moved into a small, one-story home in that city. Third grade loomed. I have no memories about being in a classroom at that school, except one. I was leaning against the fence enclosing the black asphalt playground. The sun shimmered off the surface. All the other children were on the equipment, running, throwing balls, screeching—the expected playground scene. I felt apart and different. I was unable to initiate any engagement with the group, wishing someone else would do so.

By contrast, Tim was outgoing. He even had a girlfriend who he would meet walking to school. They would fling an arm around the other's shoulder and walk on. To this day it is a source of amusement for him to ask if I remember her name. Yes, I do—Geraldine Puffinberger. I remember this and other events outside the classroom. For example, dad used to make house calls in Chinatown. I accompanied him one weekend morning. When he entered the house, a child about my age came out and sat on the stairwell beside me. No words were exchanged, but I remember being intrigued in a childlike way by this little person whose appearance and dress were unlike mine. For dad, negotiating a path between Chinese folk beliefs/remedies and Western medicine could not have been easy.

The motivation to try to put the family back together had to have been convoluted. The chance for success, particularly in San Francisco, then a magnet for the gay community, were dismal. Indeed, about half-way into the school year it was evident it would not work. Mother and the three of us left San Francisco and again relocated to grandfather's basement in Denver.

Entering school at the half year mark proved difficult. Again, my mind went elsewhere. I wasn't getting the assignments and was too timid to ask what I should be doing. It was evident others were working and I should be as well. The internal tension was great, and to relieve this I was either humming or making some utterance which drew the ire of the teacher. She warned that if this happened again I would be put out of the room. Of course it welled up, unbidden, and out to the hall I was escorted, seated on the floor, and told to stay put. Other students strolling the hall knew I had committed some egregious infraction. I was a spectacle and shamed by the experience. I remember only this singular event in the classroom. It is episodes with either strongly positive or negative valence which most readily become firmly embedded in memory. I have given thought to learning and memory. Over the long sweep of evolution, these abilities to know and store information have been integral to the development of the perceiving, thinking mind.

My maternal grandfather, George, was a rotund, bald, cheerful person who would sometimes take Tim and me to the semi-pro baseball games, a real treat. We always bet on the games. No matter the outcome, Tim and I were awarded the nickels. My grandmother, his wife, had died many years previously. I never heard about her from a family member. Grandfather had taken in his sister with dementia who rarely ventured beyond her room. When she would open her door and head toward a living room chair, mother or grandfather would quickly slip a newspaper onto the seat because of her urinary incontinence. This sister, Minnie, moved to Wyoming to homestead 160 acres of land on the eastern plains around 1895. She never married; hers must have been a hard scrabble and lonely existence. When I recently learned this history, I readily replaced my images of her in an enfeebled state with images of a brave, pioneering woman.

Dad had also left San Francisco and was living somewhere in the Denver area. One weekend morning, paying a rare, unannounced visit, he saw Tim and me playing catch in the back yard. I had practiced the exercise with the kid across the alley. We always used a hard ball. Dad picked up the ball and lofted it to me. I threw it back to Tim, who gave it to dad to throw again. With every catch the velocity increased. The old gloves we used were thin. The streaking fast balls were causing excruciating pain. Please Stop! I was silently pleading. I was unable to beg off. When he finally stopped hurling the ball I went into a secluded place in the basement and began to sob uncontrollably. Had he seen me I would have been devastated. This episode has always been hard for me to interpret, but I have a sense it encapsulated some portion of the core of our relationship.

What was he going to do with his life at this juncture, and how would this impact us? He lurched yet again. He was going to return to Rifle with us and establish his previous practice, with Marie Bell as his office nurse. Raymond Bell would be employed to complete the partially finished home we formerly occupied. Yet another attempt at reconciling the family would be made. This mercifully short experiment did not last the summer. However, before dad left we went for a horseback ride. We approached a creek, him a bit upstream, me near a waterfall where I was directed to cross. My horse bolted, and as I was departing the saddle he was able to grab my forearm as I dangled over an approximate 12-foot waterfall with rocks at the base. Memory is fragile and doesn't always serve us faithfully, but Marilyn, standing on the near bank, has often brought up this incident in conversation, verifying the details. Dad was not careful with his life or the lives of his children.

He also did not plan well and seemed to be chronically short of cash. On a trip two or three years after this horseback ride, he drove the three of us to the Teton Range in Wyoming, going on the cheap all the way. Driving back, he explained he was very low on cash, had no checks, and there were immediate needs: food, gasoline, and cigarettes. Compromises were made as we sputtered back into Rifle.

Dad moved back across the mountains to Boulder where he had found employment with the Student Health Center at the University of Colorado, a fortunate match for him. He was employed there from 1952 to 1968. The Center director and some of his colleagues were emotionally supportive. One of the nurses helped him greatly through many crises, mainly, I would assume, by listening. I surmise she was the only one he told about his sexual orientation. The students were rarely very sick, and many sought help for mental issues. Dad considered himself an astute and sensitive counselor.

Several years into this employment he decided he was going to become a psychiatrist. He was granted a three-year leave to pursue the specialty, I assume with the understanding he would come back to the Student Health Center following his training. He was accepted into the VA residency affiliated with the University of Colorado Medical School in Denver. Alas, this undertaking ended after only a year, and he was accepted back to his former employment. I recall my medical school classmates used to joke that those entering this specialty did so to try to get help for their own psychiatric maladies. This, of course, demeans the majority of such practitioners who are stable and competent, but in my dad's case this assertion may have held.

When dad left Rifle for the last time in 1952, mother gathered us in the kitchen nook with uncomfortably close spacing for "the talk." Over the previous tumultuous years, she had said nothing, at least nothing that registered. She announced in a subdued voice they were divorcing. Divorce was uncommon in those days, but I perceived enough to know that the separation was permanent. I did not know another child whose parents were divorced. I wanted to be anywhere else and heard nothing further. When she encouraged questions, I bolted for the outdoors. I stopped in the driveway. It was an overcast day. I glanced toward the Book Cliffs, repository of coveted oil trapped in shale rock. It took an effort to focus the scene. Even at this young age I had a dread that this was going to be hard, and I had compounded the difficulty by cutting myself off from a source of support, my mother, something neither of my sibs did. Of course I wondered, as many children would, what I had done to cause or contribute to this rupture. Mother never mentioned the subject again and I sure did not broach it. I sensed an emotional curtain had dropped on that day.

A day or two later I distinctly remember Tim saying to me, "now you are a bastard." I don't know where he heard this word or whether he knew that it meant, in this context, without a father. Everyone deals with pain in his/her own way. At times following the divorce, through the thin walls separating our bedrooms, I would hear Tim crying, telling mother his legs hurt. They may have hurt, but I suspect his tears were at least partially motivated by other factors. I say this because Tim is one of the most stoic people I have known, even as a child.

So, it was Rifle where we would live and continue schooling. This town has been consequential in the history of western Colorado. Though I offer only a few details, I have learned much about the history of the town from two sources: *Rifle Shots: Story of Rifle, Colorado*, self-published by a remarkable group of women who called themselves the Rifle Reading Club, and *Rifle Vignettes*, a collection of stories about the town and its residents, first published as weekly installments in the local paper by a classmate of Tim's, Betty Clifford. The Rifle Reading Club organized in 1903 with the stated goals of 1) mutual improvement, 2) to learn about social affairs, and 3) to help each other to a better understanding of state and national affairs. The club's motto was: "No excellence without labor." They founded the first public library shortly after their formation, and over the years fostered many civic-minded activities. They lobbied diligently to allow women to vote in Colorado. After a century in existence, the Rifle Reading Club disbanded.

Rifle is in a valley, about a mile in elevation, rimmed by hills, mesas, and higher mountains in the distance. The indigenous inhabitants of this valley, the Utes, were vanquished in 1879 at the Meeker Massacre, and in 1881 were placed on reservations. The land they occupied was sold by the government, attracting settlers from all quadrants of the nation. The majority was seeking permanence and stability, a plot of land to graze livestock on the high plateaus and raise feed, crops, and fruit. Some were the unlucky migrants chasing the get-rich-quick lure of gold, silver, and lead. These early settlers would not have predicted that Rifle would be the center of a future rush, this to extract the billions of barrels of potential oil from the shale rock in the Book Cliffs and similar formations extending into Utah. The Colorado River separates the main portion of the town from dwellings (and now businesses) across the river. A railroad line runs parallel to the river. The first line was established in 1889, linking Rifle to passenger service. It became a major hub, transporting livestock and produce, and bringing in supplies. Among the railway workers were Hispanics. Their descendants were well integrated into the school system and its culture when I was growing up.

The highlight of early existence in Rifle was a 1905 speech by President Theodore Roosevelt on a platform erected adjacent to a small blue schoolhouse on Divide Creek, 17 miles from Rifle. Every available form of transportation ferried over 1,000 people to see and hear their beloved leader. Rifle and surrounding areas were empty on that day. Roosevelt was there to hunt bear and was camped a few miles away. He rode over the crest of a hill on a white horse, unaccompanied by anyone, wearing his canvas hunting outfit and white Stetson hat. His rapt audience, having finished their picnics and decked in their finest, waved red, white, and blue handkerchiefs. He gave a speech titled: "Success—What it Means." Beautifully written accounts recorded this event. Four years earlier Roosevelt and his party had stayed at the Winchester Hotel in Rifle on route to hunt mountain lions near Meeker, just up the road from Rifle.

The idyllic scene at the school stood in contrast to the unrest to come. Oil shale was discovered about the time the Utes were driven off the land. Subsequently the government made a few tentative explorations. When oil and gas were in short supply during WWII, these efforts increased. The Navy established the Naval Oil Reserve and built a small town, Anvil Points, eight miles west of Rifle. It was an attractive community of scientists and workers, built from prefabricated materials. Some of the children were very bright, setting a high bar for the rest of us. I remember a visit to the community. They had their own basketball court, ice rink, and a small movie theatre. By the early to mid-1950s the funding for the project dwindled. The efforts to recover shale oil had not, however, ended.

After third grade in San Francisco and Denver, during which I was mentally absent and learned very little, the Denver school recommended that I repeat third grade. That would have been a major emotional setback. Two women became my advocates. The fourth-grade teacher, Mrs. Mary Ammerman, a woman of large frame and larger heart, in consultation with her higher ups and mother, sought to defy this recommendation. She prevailed and I entered fourth grade in her class.

Though dad had moved to Boulder, Marie and Raymond remained in Rifle for a short period before they also moved. Marie knew I had fallen woefully behind in school and worked with me on basic math, using a homemade bean bag. She would provide the two numbers for addition or subtraction, throw the bag, and I was to attempt an answer before catching it. With these efforts on the part of these caring women I slowly got back on track. So much intellectual capital is squandered when children fall behind and are not afforded the resources I had. Tim seemed to have taken his disrupted second year of school in stride, but lurking below the surface was a major disability, dyslexia, which he has dealt with over the years through Herculean determination and effort.

Following Mrs. Ammerman, several other teachers were excellent and innovative. Mrs. Esma Lewis had taught in several nearby small towns before settling in Rifle permanently. It would not be enough to say she was invested in student learning. I once recall her brought to tears by a recalcitrant student whose defenses she could not penetrate. Though her display could be thought unseemly, it does convey the depth of her commitment. She won many teaching awards in the valley and was listed in Who's Who in Elementary Education. The local elementary school was named in her honor.

Ms. Nancy Lester, the sixth-grade teacher, was energetic and inspired. She began the morning class by leading restless and reluctant pupils in singing rounds, the class initially divided in half, then into thirds when we improved. The result, as I recall it today, was stunning. After weeks of this routine willing, even eager, students began to relish the singing. As discordant notes were purged, harmony ultimately prevailed. This exercise seemed to wonderfully focus the mind. Following this ritual, the class was more attentive and ready to learn. Before coming to Rifle Ms. Lester had written a whimsical novel about an east coast college graduate hired to teach in a small town between Rifle and Aspen.[5] The stories had an autobiographical cast about them.

Over these years, despite more success in school and largely helpful teachers, I remained withdrawn, reticent, easily wounded by perceived slights, and always on guard that I not give offense. I countered these traits by becoming very competitive. Achieving good grades, better than my peers, became a goal apart from learning. The competitive sphere of athletics also consumed me; baseball in the summer, football and basketball beginning in the seventh grade. Becoming immersed in scholarship and athletics was a partially successful antidote to distracted, inner-directed thinking. Interspersed, occasionally, amongst the jumble of these other mental activities was scary contemplation of such weighty subjects as Nothingness and Infinity, intrusive mental outliers which have bedeviled scientists, philosophers, and theologians for eons. A lot of ink has been spilled in trying to explicate these bookends of existential dread.

Television arrived relatively late in Rifle. This meant outdoor activities; summer afternoons at the local reservoir and hiking in the nearby hills in search of arrowheads. That left ample time for other activities. The neighborhood was populated by teenagers older than me, some of whom were creative pranksters and activity organizers. One of the colorful characters was Robert (Bob) Collett, six years older than me. On a flat stretch of ground near the rivulet below our house he built a pig pen. When one of his sows was heavily pregnant and due soon, he gathered his peers in the neighborhood to sleep out near the pen in case his pet sow might need help during delivery. He offhandedly offered me the chance to join in this important work, so important that the neighborhood female teenagers were expected to bring us food at night. On the second morning of this vigil, we awoke to witness the sow lying on her side, contentedly nursing her healthy offspring. Bob subsequently became a veterinarian, moved to California to establish a practice, and held numerous positions of leadership among his veterinary fraternity.

Another older neighbor used his connection to pigs to become a top-notch runner. John Fennell was sickly as a child but became one of the premier milers in the state by running several miles a day on a country road to feed his pigs. He and my brother were two of the most disciplined and resolute people I have known. John ascended the ranks in the DuPont Company as an agricultural researcher. He had an abiding interest in history, particularly Civil War history. After years of painstaking research, he wrote the Civil War and post-war histories of 290 soldiers who graduated in the lowest quartile of their West Point Academy classes,[6] a book intended as a reference source. He was able to fully document lives of all but one soldier. This group was overrepresented in the ranks of battlefield generals and leaders, including General George Custer. They were, as his research showed, "better warriors than students." He dedicated the volume to a soldier who had clearly suffered from PTSD, and he urged that more war historians call attention to this malady. The last time I saw John he was in his 80s and beginning another book.

While often not directly germane, neighbors, schoolmates, teachers, and mentors may add context to anyone's narrative. In this light, another neighborhood family lived across the dirt alleyway separating our houses. The father published the weekly Rifle Telegram. The youngest of three children, a son, was an unapologetic homosexual during the era this identity could get one shunned or worse. Following college, K. C. worked in the active bath houses of Denver at a time HIV and hepatitis B were ravaging the gay community. He learned that the University of Colorado Medical School was conducting trials to determine the safety and efficacy of an experimental hepatitis B vaccine. He recruited a large cadre of volunteers from his place of employment to participate in these ultimately successful experiments. This important development came, alas, too late for dad. I will forever see a deep connection between dad and that gangly, uncompromising kid with curly red hair.

Many youngsters in the neighborhood had jobs. When I was 11 and 12, I had a morning newspaper route, delivering one of the two Denver papers. In addition to delivery, I was responsible for the monthly collections. The job paid a pittance, but the only way to get this meager amount was to knock on doors for the monthly collection, an aspect of the job which required the dreaded "asking" for something. Occasionally, after knocking, I would see a curtain part and close again, but no answer at the door. Rifle was hilly. One

Sunday morning I had unrolled the canvas bags strung over the handlebars until they touched the ground, the only way the papers with the Sunday supplements could be accommodated. I was starting at the top of one of the steeper hills. The bike had one gear and no chain guard. As I rode down the hill with the bags skimming the road, the metal band wrapped around the lower portion of the pants leg slipped over my ankle and the inevitable occurred. The loose material caught between the chain and the sprocket, the bike abruptly pitched forward, and I went over the handlebars. Many of the papers and their innards were scattered at the scene and down the hill. I hardly noticed the abrasions in the urgency to extricate myself from the chain, reassemble the papers, and get back on the road.

Unless we motored over the passes (no tunnels through the mountains at that time) at Christmas to stay with mother's relatives, as was expected, we rarely saw my father. He would make an appearance on Christmas day. I was old enough to be acutely aware of the forced harmony. These holidays were sad, but there was never an expectation on my part they would be otherwise. More promising were visits to the Rye log cabin in the summer. I held out the hope he would make the effort to be just a regular dad. However, whenever Tim and I were summoned to Rye, it became evident the main reason was always an onerous project that needed doing. One time it was digging a hole for a new outdoor latrine. On another occasion we were to hand-saw logs for firewood. When we went to Rye as younger children, dad's mother was still alive. She would sit on the porch, smoke cigarettes, and listen to professional baseball games on the radio. She was intolerant of any loud noises, and made it known.

I recall with clarity an episode at the Rye cabin when I was a youngster. It was midafternoon and I was lying on a bed resting after assigned "chores." Dad opened the door and lay next to me without uttering a word. He reached out and placed a hand on my thigh. It was not sexual (he rarely touched his children), but I became acutely uncomfortable. He stared at the ceiling. At that time I was unfamiliar with the term depression and its manifestations, but the air was thick with, what, unhappiness? His state of mind seemed to exude a thick layer of almost palpable gloom. Much later I learned that he was hospitalized and received electroconvulsive therapy, though I do not know when. Was it near this point in his life? If not, I now wonder how much lower he could have sunk until something would have to be done.

A brief detour is warranted at this juncture. The memories or vignettes chosen for this narrative may seem somewhat random. It is my wish that those I have selected to write about may add perspective, even if somewhat peripheral, for the upcoming science chapters. Several friends who have read this material have opined that dredging up these snippets may hearken back to time in a therapist's office, time not always productively spent. They have questioned that perhaps this writing attempt is, at least partially, another effort to reframe the past. Whatever the motivation, memories have always been a means to tell a story and will undergird this one.

Another summer dad had plans for Tim and me in a community other than Rye. Because he worked at a college, he could arrange summers off when student numbers were low. He leased a hamburger stand in George-town, Colorado, and converted it to the Hi-Ho Café with about four to six tables. Tim and I were going to bus tables, do dishes, and clean up. Dad would take orders and cook the food. It became quickly evident this was another failed enterprise, and after only two days he went back to Boulder, and we returned to Rifle. This, at least, allowed me to resume summer baseball.

A year following the Hi-Ho Café debacle, dad signed on to be the head wrangler at a summer camp in the foothills 10 miles outside Boulder. The three of us joined him. For me, this proved to be the most beneficial decision he ever made. Tim and I returned to the camp four additional summers, and Marilyn an additional two summers. The standard camp activities of horseback riding, archery, crafts, water sports, and other activities were offered. Trojan Ranch also supported gymnastics. Don Robinson, the coach of a suburban Denver high school team, ran the gymnastics program. He was dedicated and reliable. The camp director transferred many duties to his broad shoulders in addition to gymnastics. He had competed in college gymnastics, and thereafter dedicated his life to the sport and the athletes fortunate to have him as their coach. He was also expert at tooling leather and creating other artwork, the majority of which he generously gave away.

Don was one of the most decent persons I have known. He remembers being left in the back seat of a car to sleep while his parents were in a bar. His care was ultimately transferred to grandparents. He eschewed all harmful substances. He was sensitive to others with troubled upbringings. On some nights after lights-out, he would suggest he, another camper whose parents had divorced when he was young, and me accompany him on a hike up to the remnants of an old fire lookout station overlooking the lights of Boulder below and Denver in the distance. He understood emotional pain and was not reluctant to talk about it. He had faced it down and, with uncompromising courage, became the ultimate positive role model. He treated us like adults, encouraging any verbalization we wished to share. I wanted to be in his company as much as possible. For the latter two of the five years I attended this camp, I was a counselor and accompanied my younger charges when they went to their assigned morning and afternoon activities. But I freed up as much time as I could manage to "help out" with the gymnastics program. Don worked with me because I showed aptitude and desire on the tumbling mats and trampoline.

Another Rifle alumnus had a surprising tie to Don. Charles (Chuck) Jones was six years ahead of me in school. He went to Colorado State College in Greeley where he inexplicably became interested in gymnastics. As a result, he became a friend of Don's who, at that time, was a member of the college's gymnastics team. Chuck took up trampoline, and on a visit to Rifle contacted me with an invitation to accompany him to a trampoline park in Grand Junction, 60 miles away. These parks were generally populated by frivolity seeking youngsters. This was not the intent of Chuck Jones. He was there for a strenuous workout. Though I did not know him well, I became quickly aware he was a driven individual. His subsequent career in the Air Force bears this out. He flew B52 bombers, and later became Commander at three Air Force Bases. I visited him later in life at his residence in Dayton, Ohio, home of the Wright Patterson Air Force Base. A concrete bench memorializing his service and referencing the bases he commanded is on the grounds of the museum accompanying Wright Patterson.

A major event in Rifle is the annual Garfield County Fair and Rodeo, with a parade down the main streets of the town. Parade entries of all descriptions were welcome. Chuck suggested we invite Don to showcase gymnastics. Don would go to great lengths to promote the sport he loved, and readily consented. He also was a bit of a showman, in addition to his other qualities. A trampoline was placed on a flat-bed truck and maneuvers performed as the parade moved forward. Don suggested a trick from summer camp days. I was in a handstand atop his outstretched frame when the tops of my pointed toes clipped a heretofore unseen wire crossing the street. We came down in a heap on the trampoline bed. I doubt this was a scene Don would have selected to promote his sport.

Don became the gymnastics coach at Arizona State University. In 1986 I was driving through Nebraska after a medical meeting. I had remembered the college gymnastics finals were to be in Omaha that weekend. The timing was right. A friend and I attended the final evening. It came down to the final event, but ASU won the national championship by a slim margin. Arizona State had been runners-up in 1974 and 1978 under his leadership. I was invited to the post-victory celebration at a local restaurant. I sensed the admiration and warmth the athletes (and particularly their parents in attendance) had for Don. He pointed me out to the crowd and spoke a few kind words. I recall a rush of emotion, somewhat reminiscent of feelings at summer camp when, hands clasped, he would swing me between his legs, up over his head, whereupon I would unfurl into a handstand (as I had during our ill-fated parade performance). This represented, for me, an elemental bond with this fine man. Don was the first recipient of the USA Gymnastics Lifetime Achievement Award in 2000. Years later I tried to contact him and was greatly saddened to learn he had died.

Summer camp provided me some needed socialization. However, when the school year resumed, I would lapse back into what was becoming a familiar pattern; competing to get good grades and devoting time and effort to sports competition. Moving to the ninth grade, high school, was a big adjustment. It had always been a challenge for me to fit in, but now there was the prospect of social engagement on a truly awkward scale. The upperclassmen had swagger and seeming confidence, pairing off in relationships I craved but deemed unattainable. Had I been a little more open to friendship and communication, I would doubtless have sensed I was not alone in feeling the way I did.

Looming like a Leviathan was the "new" football program. A year prior to my entering high school a head coach was hired, Gordon Cooper, who had played professional football for the Detroit Lions. In his senior year in college, he caught more passes than any other player in the country. He enjoyed hunting and the outdoors; Rifle amply provided an outlet for these passions. He brought a tough mindset to grueling practices. Long, full pad scrimmages were punishing. Most of us were pressed into service to complete an offense and defense. As a freshman defensive back, blockers and runners more than twice my size would barrel toward me with no intention of easing up. I was getting pummeled. I had more than a few Please Stop! moments, as I had when dad hurled hard balls at me in Denver. Our practice and game field was home to a rodeo only weeks before the start of the season, the Garfield County Fair and Rodeo. It was, thus, a decidedly unhygienic turf. There was also hazing by upperclassmen. Some of it directed toward a few of my classmates in the locker room was extreme and perverse. To his credit, when the coach found out how far out of bounds this had become, he ended the most egregious violations. One evening after practice, mother noticed I was more morose than usual. She asked the reason, and I offered a small hint. Though I am sure she was conflicted, in her own soft way she encouraged me to stick it out. In that short exchange, the emotional curtain I had dropped was raised just a little.

Gordon Cooper could deliver praise and blistering criticism in equal measure. I recall (and cringe when I do) some of his rhetoric in the latter category. He was usually measured, but his face would redden and spittle would form at the corners of his mouth as he exhorted a better performance. The players respected him and put forth great effort. In our senior season the team tied for the state championship in our division (ties were not resolved back then). I was the quarterback behind a very beefy and mobile line.

One sport I truly enjoyed was basketball and was a starter in eighth grade. In the first year of high school I was on the junior varsity team, but never saw playing time. The following winter I opted to join the wrestling team rather than spend another season potentially on the bench. The decision was a bit impulsive. I had never wrestled, though had a sense of the steep learning curve and the physical and mental commitment the sport requires if one was to do well. The coach was Gordon Cooper, the demanding football coach. Though he learned the sport on the job, he was a quick study. He knew good physical conditioning was essential; there were no short cuts. I committed to the rigor. I carefully watched the team's model student-athlete, Stan Snyder, three years my senior. He was a leader by example who offered his own brand of quiet encouragement. Stan was Rifle's first state champion. He later obtained a Veterinary degree and became a professor on faculty at the Oregon State University School of Veterinary Medicine. Toward the end of the first season, I began to improve and win a few matches.

For the final two years I would do what was required to win, including the grueling weight loss to drop to the lowest weight class possible, as many of my competitors were doing. Fortunately, today there are regulations which prevent extreme, unhealthy weight loss.

Tim wrestled his freshman and sophomore years and was a starter as a sophomore. Both of us were shedding weight, pounds early in the week after a weekend of gorging, and then ounces as the weigh-in for the next match neared. Mother was adamant we should eat and aggrieved when her proffered food was barely touched. Toward the end of a week of intense dieting we hatched a plan. We would funnel the rations to the pet dog, Sooner, positioned under the table. After only a few days this ruse was spotted. These were halcyon days for this mutt while they lasted. This is the only time I recall mother crying. I saw the tears welling, then she turned away—I don't even recall tears at dad's funeral, though I did not necessarily scrutinize for this effect. We were taking away a reason for her existence, to provide basic care and comfort.

This dog was the selfsame one who offered my first glimpse into the emotional life and memory of an animal. A bridge over the Colorado River was crossed to get to the town's veterinarian. The dog often went on excursions in the car with us, never crossing the river unless for the occasional visit to the vet. One day, with mother driving, Tim alongside, and me in the back seat with the dog, we made the turn onto the bridge. This signaled only one thing; we were going to the vet. The dog started gasping, almost wheezing, intermittently laying on its back, emitting pitiful, faint, bark-like exhalations. This "attack" was quite a production. I will address this issue of emotional memory in mammals when I bring more basic science to the subject in later chapters.

A few years later I could empathize with the dog, though in a less demonstrative way. If I or someone else was a few ounces short of the mark for a wrestling match weigh in, we would often resort to being rolled up in small mats, arms to the side, to sweat off the remaining ounces. While I was thus cocooned, someone sat on the rolled-up mat and wouldn't get off despite my initial entreaties to do so. The anxiety rose, leading to a panic attack, a most dreadful sense of uncontrollable terror despite the absence of a real threat. Once this was underway, I endured it silently until the offender got up and wandered off. As I later reflected, this was the first time I learned my physiology had a trigger, a set point beyond which this full body reaction would manifest, a set point likely much lower than the average.

I had successful junior and senior wrestling seasons, advancing to the state tournament in Denver both years, and winning a state championship my senior year. Boulder was just up the road. Though I did not expect he would be there, I quickly, almost unconsciously, scanned the crowd when coming off the mat for the last time. My hard work would have been validated by dad's presence. I don't think he ever knew I won a state title. It was during these years mother was almost housebound. She did come to one wrestling meet in Rifle but was unable to stay for my match. She made the effort; I never thought less of her. Despite (or maybe because of) the grind and sacrifices, wrestling became, for me, a template for slogging through future difficulties, even if this template operated largely beneath the surface of consciousness.

Dad's absence at the wrestling tournament was trivial when I think about Tim and his struggles (though I don't think this is a word he would use). In high school he was confronted with challenges which would wither most mortals. In addition to severe dyslexia, he began to experience back pain. X-rays showed degenerative changes in his lower back. He had wrestled and played football in ninth and tenth grades but was advised against further participation in these sports. This was tough, but he faced both the learning, and now physical, difficulties with a quiet determination. He was given exercises he was allowed. He developed his own regimen around these recommendations, doing a prodigious amount of exercise, ultimately sculpting a body I would not want to face on a wrestling mat. This same drive and determination animated his studies with equally striking results. It took all available hours of the day and many at night, in addition to sheer perseverance and stamina, to excel when his ability to read, write, and spell were so compromised. When he could no longer participate in sports, he became equipment manager, meaning he was assigned any job the coaches needed doing. I recall football practice concentrated at one end of the field, looking toward the other end and seeing Tim seated on the ground under the goal post with books spread before him, ever ready to leave this post and discharge any duties given him.

Despite his dyslexia, he was always a logical and deep thinker, always able to make cogent arguments and defend a stance. We all have learning strengths and liabilities. Fortunately, Tim was born with neural circuits that favored math, physics, mechanical abilities, and related subjects. It must be mentioned that Tim got an A in every course in high school. This was unprecedented in my memory, though this feat is likely to have happened before our time in school and repeated since. With all this, Tim managed an active social life. I do not remember a time in high school he did not have a girlfriend. He was also adventurous. After high school graduation he toured Europe on a motorcycle, staying in hostels and making friends along the way. He financed his trip by working several summers with a surveyor. Later in life he learned to SCUBA dive and skied on glaciers in Canada, ferried to the top in helicopters.

Tim, Marilyn, and I are indebted to many Rifle high school teachers in addition to those in the lower grades. To this pantheon Marilyn would later be added, though she went through her own travails with aplomb, resilience, and a sense of purpose before she became a high school teacher in the Rifle school system. We had a varied group of teachers, as would be expected, but some deserve mention. Mr. Coston Cerise, the high school basketball coach, was a modest man and a superb math teacher. He assigned Tim and a student-athlete in my class, David Peercy, harder math problems not in the texts, taking time to work with these gifted students. David, valedictorian of the class, was also a musician (piano and clarinet) of considerable talent and was the fullback on our football team. He went on to letter twice in football and three times in track at the University of Colorado, earn a PhD in mathematics, and have a distinguished career in various government laboratories. Despite all his accomplishments, Dave would likely regard his 13 years on the Albuquerque School Board as the most consequential. For five of these years, he was the elected president. Given Dave's relentless pursuit of excellence, I know a curriculum change or alteration in teaching methods would have to be supported by solid data to receive his support. He found himself at odds with the views on education espoused by the extant state government. In a stark example of politicization of the electoral process, the governor and her staff issued a robocall in one of the elections advocating a no-vote against Dave. He won that election for school board president overwhelmingly.

Some of the more liberal teachers in Rifle held views that were not congruent with those of the generally conservative town folk. A history teacher, Ms. Ann Gavin, sometimes betrayed her views in the classroom. During the Cuban missile crisis, she was vocal in her concern. She was labeled alarmist by some, though she was correct in her assessment that the brinkmanship during this crisis could (and nearly did) precipitate a nuclear war. She had learned that a law still on the books, though not enforced, forbade a black from remaining in town after sunset. She railed against this. By dress, mannerisms, and speech, she was not mainstream. Some of us were attracted to her views, which seemed fringe and just a little dangerous to others. If she was the harbinger of the hippie culture to come, she was certainly one of the more responsible proponents of this view of life.

An English teacher also tested the limits of acceptability. He thought we should be exposed to J. D. Salinger's *Catcher in the Rye*. Though tame by today's standards, it was on the banned list of books we were to be shielded from. He began to read the book aloud in class. The school principal heard of this transgression and threatened a firing. The English teacher persisted and was summarily fired. With nothing to lose, he continued every day reading to the class, and every day the principal stood in the doorway, arms folded across his chest, glowering. It was a standoff with no clear winner. The book was read through, and the teacher left town at the end of the school year.

Another teacher, responsible for directing the junior-senior class play, selected *The Glass Menagerie* by Tennessee Williams. It was a somewhat audacious pick for a small western Colorado community. It was not typical of plays staged in Rifle. In many fundamental ways the play reflects the life of the brilliant but troubled author.[7] I was surprised and unsure when the teacher selected me to be one of the four actors: a narrator (me), the narrator's sister, their mother, and a gentleman calling on the sister. This complex drama was emotionally layered, staged in a single living room and accompanying alleyway. Looming on the fireplace mantle was a picture of the largely absent father. The narrator was detached, vaguely alienated, striving to find identity and a mission. In contrast to my role in the second grade Peter Cottontail play in which I tossed a carrot across the stage at the wrong time, I felt oddly comfortable and identified with this role. All four actors, including David Peercy as the gentleman caller, delivered their lines flawlessly and were emotionally true to their characters. The large audience seemed genuinely appreciative. My role allowed expression I had previously submerged, and I realized I had some emotional "juice." But back into the interior it slinked.

The play brings to mind the memory of another, unrelated scene from years earlier. The main stage was at the end of the junior high basketball court. One noon in junior high I was urged to join two or three older boys for a smoke in a hidden area of the wooden edifice over the stage. I succumbed to the pressure and hesitantly joined, feigned a practiced air, and snuffed the butt into the wooden beams as I witnessed them do. That night I was unable to sleep, waiting for the wail of the fire engine siren on the way to the burning school.

The play was a brief, but meaningful interlude. There were grades to be earned, sports goals to be conquered, and "leadership" to exercise. If I was not in the mix socially, this behavior did not prevent my election to junior class president and student body president as a senior. It seemed good grades, athletics, and a non-controversial persona was the margin. I was utterly bereft as a leader at that time. The anonymity of a big city school would have rescued me. I was unable to forcefully push an agenda or to lean on someone to do a job (I would rather do it myself). Getting enough students to participate in a car wash required personal intervention, which I would do only as a last resort. I largely avoided any conflict, which leaders cannot do. However, conflict and competition which were structured and sanctioned, like athletics, was an acceptable outlet.

If leadership proved difficult for me, a student in Tim's class, a year behind him in high school, assumed the mantle of leadership with an ease I have rarely witnessed, as if born to it. Russell George was a genuinely friendly individual who obviously liked his fellow humans. In high school he was elected to the posts I held and more. After graduating from Harvard Law School, he returned to Rifle, his life-long residence, and was for many years a state legislator, serving as Speaker of the House for two years. He was later appointed director of the Colorado Division of Wildlife and executive director of the Colorado Department of Natural Resources under both Democratic and Republican governors. In 2018 he received the Citizenship Medal from the governor. In Iowa City I attended a political fundraiser featuring Diana DeGette, a Colorado U.S. House of Representatives member, as the main speaker. I was involved with stem cell research at the time, and, knowing her strong advocacy for the field, I engaged her on this topic following her speech. I also indicated I was from Colorado. What town, she inquired? She beamed when I answered Rifle, asking if I knew Russell. She, a Democrat, emphasized how often he (a Republican) pushed for bipartisanship when both were in the Colorado legislature.

Another Republican lawmaker from Rifle, in marked contrast to Russell George, has symbolized the bitterly partisan politics of recent times. Lauren Boebert was elected to the House of Representatives from the 3rd Congressional district in 2020. When she and her husband moved to the area in 2013, they opened a restaurant called Shooters Grille. She wore a loaded pistol and encouraged the wait staff to do likewise. This stance in support of the second amendment to the Constitution attracted national attention. She was interviewed by numerous national news outlets at the time. My curiosity aroused, I went to peer through the restaurant window when I was in Rifle visiting my sister. A waitress, no doubt accustomed to gawkers, glanced my way and coyly smiled. As I write this shortly after the Capitol invasion on January 6, 2021, Representative Boebert has attempted to defy the prohibition against bringing firearms to Congress.

At some point during junior high a family of five moved into the basement and the four of us moved into the upstairs Raymond Bell had completed. The chance to escape to an isolated corner of the house was precluded. It was cramped and was going to get a little more so. I got my first hint of Marilyn's pregnancy when Kenny, her boyfriend, was ribbed in the locker room about becoming a daddy. There was confirmation when the physical manifestations became obvious. I watched with something approaching curiosity as she continued to grow bigger. She went to class as long as feasible. The school principal volunteered to provide home assignments and grade them so she could graduate with her class. Imagine! She delivered a boy before graduation. A small wedding ceremony followed later that year. Dad came over and, at least in my presence, assumed the role of a wronged parent. He would be unaware of this rank hypocrisy. Mother did what she could to help my sister. I saw no evidence she was judgmental or scolding.

Kenny's life, apart from school sports, revolved around rodeo, hunting, and my sister. Marilyn was outgoing and popular, with a close circle of friends. They started dating early in high school. This gave me entre into a social sphere and activities I would not otherwise have been privy to. Though three years older than me, Kenny and his friends allowed me to accompany them when they traveled to rodeos and on deer hunting trips. My sensibilities did not mesh easily with this culture, but their acceptance of my presence was a validation of sorts. Kenny competed in most events on the rodeo grounds; bareback and saddle bronc riding, bull riding, team and individual roping events, and garnered many prizes (gaudy belt buckles, trophies, etc.). Peer pressure and conformity on these trips was a burden against which I had little resistance. Beer was a staple. I was perhaps 13 on the first outing. Imbibing this fluid produced a predictable train of responses; giddiness, euphoria, and strings of idiotic verbalizations, followed in turn by sickness and the other depredations of too much alcohol.

On one deer hunting trip Kenny, two of his friends, and I drove in Kenny's doorless, old jeep to the top of the Book Cliffs along a narrow road. Coming off the mountain in the dark, having negotiated the switchbacks, Kenny rounded a less challenging turn at a high rate of speed. When the wheels struck the gravel on the side of the road the jeep flipped, sending Kenny and friends flying out, sustaining non-serious injuries. I was straddling the gear shift, which I probably instinctively grabbed. The vehicle rolled over and over, first a glimpse of the canvas top, then of the floor, iterated many times. Aside from a few abrasions, I was not injured.

Kenny was one tough human. In football practice early in the season his senior year he badly dislocated his elbow. A cast was placed. There was a question if he would play the remainder of the year. He watched one game from the sidelines, had his cast removed, played out the year, and became an all-state guard. He was offered a football scholarship to a small college, but he was not really college material and was undersized. He got a job with a company drilling cores from the earth to determine if mining operations (mostly copper) might prove to be profitable. For eight years they were on the move; Colorado, New Mexico, Arizona, Utah, Michigan, and Puerto Rico, initially with one child, but soon thereafter a daughter was born. Most of their time was spent in trailer parks.

Ultimately, they got back to Colorado where Kenny was able to become more involved with horses and ranching operations and Marilyn attended a junior college. When they moved to Livermore, about a 25-mile drive from Ft. Collins, she commuted to Colorado State University and completed her degree. When they moved back to Rifle, she was hired by the high school from which she had graduated to teach Vocational Business. In addition, she was sponsor for the Future Business Leaders of America. One of her students became national vice president of this organization. She also initiated Mock Trial on the entire Western slope of Colorado after she had witnessed these competitions in Denver. She convinced her superiors of their learning benefit and arranged Colorado Bar Association sponsorship. Kenny, meantime, had numerous jobs, including packing hunters into the high country to pursue elk (with Marilyn as cook when she was able) as well as leading wild horse roundups in Nevada, funded by the Bureau of Land Management. The horses were offered for adoption.

When walking the halls of the high school, I would occasionally glance into the office of the superintendent, Lafayette ("Lefty") Green, who always left the door open. He seemed to have a perpetual scowl. I often thought I would not want to be sent to his office. It was only later in life, when I was in the Navy, that I was fortunate to get to know this warm, caring gentleman after he persuaded my mother, then doing better emotionally and working as his secretary, to marry him. His wife died years before in a car accident in which Lefty was the driver. I have been grateful that mother was able to spend her remaining seven years in this mutually supportive relationship. I escaped for several weeks to a small space in their basement of their home in Rifle following the breakup of a relationship and the start of a career in Iowa.

After my graduation (53 students) in 1962, Rifle witnessed several events which made national, and even international, news after I left for college. The first such event attracted widespread attention in 1969. Natural gas, locked in geologic deposits, could be an alternative to oil, or could supplement oil production. With advice and consent of the Atomic Energy Commission and commercial backing of two companies, a hole over 8,000 feet deep was dug at Rulison, seven miles southwest of Rifle. A forty-kiloton bomb, twice the explosive power as that dropped on Hiroshima, was placed in the hole. It was reasoned that vast amounts of natural gas would collect in a huge holding chamber which could be distributed for energy needs. The government assured residents it was safe. Following the detonation, there was some damage to buildings nearby, but more importantly the gas which was collected could not be used because it was radioactive. Several other smaller bombs were detonated near Rifle with the same result.[8]

The second scenario to garner attention was a further attempt at oil shale development which had ceased when Anvil Points was closed. However, with the OPEC oil embargo of the late 1970s, it again appeared that a profit could feasibly be made from the extraction of oil from shale rock. The government leased over 5,000 acres of land to oil companies; the most dominant was Exxon Mobil. As Betty Clifford noted in *Rifle Vignettes*, the *New York Times* wrote of a small town (Rifle) of 2,200 people "who left doors unlocked, shook hands on business deals, and often left keys in cars. They were innocents who didn't have a clue about what was coming." It was predicted the population could top 20,000 by 1990. The population did swell rapidly to about 12,000 when, by the vagaries of market forces, Exxon precipitously pulled out on May 2, 1982 (known locally as Black Sunday) and locked the gates. This saga exemplifies the history of boom-and-bust cycles of shale oil extraction.[9] More durable for Rifle had been its long history of vanadium mining and processing. This element, used to harden steel, was much in demand during WWII. Subsequently, the tailings from vanadium processing were an important source of uranium. As children we played on these tailings up Rifle Creek.

More benign, but also attracting international attention, was the 1971 offering by the artist Christo Javacheff. Christo, his preferred appellation, had gained notoriety/fame for wrapping buildings such as the Reichstag, the Parliament building in Berlin, with woven swaths of material, and for many other projects. Wealthy patrons backed his plan to hang an orange-copper curtain made of nylon polyamide from large cables bridging the road to Rifle Creek. Wind scuttled the first attempt. After adjustments, the curtain was unfurled ten months later. This wondrous spectacle was again split asunder by wind 28 hours later, not to be resurrected.

After the final winter wrestling season, I was looking forward to spring and fewer commitments. Alas, it was not to be. Coach Cooper wanted to start a junior high wrestling program. These existed at some of the competitor schools. He did not ask if I would be the coach; he assumed I would. There was no denying him. I put in long hours with these new recruits, took them to meets and one tournament. Though as a team we were not stellar, there were some promising young athletes to send on.

This telling would not be complete without mention of a wholly unexpected proposal. I only had two dates in high school, both to the junior-senior proms. I thought I was largely invisible to the opposite sex. However, in the waning months of school a classmate of notable beauty and, by reputation, experience, coyly asked if I would like to "be intimate," or words to that effect. An aroused state was quickly swamped by a competing narrative, an inner persona I had unknowingly cultivated and internalized, that of a paragon of virtue. This stance is difficult to sustain, but it held for this moment as I fumbled for a response. I finally settled on this Holy statement: that this act was best reserved for marriage. I was perplexed by my response the moment I uttered it. Would life have been different had I assented?

Yes, this encounter was memorable, but more impactful than almost any other high school event was a biology class field trip. A petite, reserved teacher, Ms. Phyllis Matheny, took the class, her microscopes in hand, to look at pond water near a small reservoir outside town. As an aside, David Peercy mentioned to me, when we relived our high school days in a conversation years later, that when Ms. Matheny strolled through practice one afternoon, someone tossed her a basketball. She put the basketball through the hoop from a significant distance, not once but several times. David knew a history about her I did not. In high school in Iowa, she was a starter on her girls' basketball team that had won a state championship. Six-girl basketball (three on offense and three on defense) was hugely popular in Iowa; the large arena in Des Moines nearly filled for some of the tournament games. I am sure Ms. Matheny was aware of the history of girls' basketball in Rifle. In the 1920s it was a major draw. For three years in a row Rifle won the western slope championship. In 1931 Colorado officials deemed the sport too strenuous for girls and ended it, not to be reinstated until 1972 with the passage of Title IX.

The slides with pond water were placed on the stage of the microscope. When I peered down the tube at the multitude of wriggling, squirming, darting organisms in this unseen world, I was enthralled. As mundane as this episode sounds, an oceanic sense of connection to life beyond the confines of our human-centric view suffused my being. It was surpassing, made more tangible by her pond-side lecture. This teacher cared about the subject matter and seemed to have a deep connection to it. I have reflected that if evolution had been taught in schools back then, Ms. Matheny would have been a compelling and powerful spokesperson to reveal the continuity of all life, beginning about 3.5 to 3.8 billion years ago with the first evidence for the appearance of bacteria. Bacteria are foundational to life on this planet. Chapter 2 is devoted to this premise.

※※※

WHEN IT was time to consider colleges, I took the advice of the trusted veterinarian in town who had obtained his degree at Colorado State University in Ft. Collins. Dad had also attended this college with the intent to become a forest ranger, but after two years he left to pursue a pre-med course at the college in Boulder. When I arrived on campus in 1962, the incoming class was provided an orientation session wherein we were to declare a major and be assigned an advisor. I was under the mistaken impression we did not have to choose a major until later in the school year. I perused the list of possible majors and selected, almost by impulse, Social Studies. At the end of the first quarter, after taking introductory Sociology, I knew I had to change majors. I went to the career counselor's office. His staff administered a battery of aptitude tests, after which he called me in and opened with the question "have you ever considered becoming a doctor?" This field scored far ahead of all others. I was taken aback. My father had let it be known in subtle ways and not so subtle language his discomfort with his profession. Given his attitude, I had likely considered that medicine was not for me. But upon taking my leave of the career counselor I went directly to the appropriate office to fill out the paperwork to switch to Physical Sciences and was assigned a new advisor.

Certainly, the most important decision was a career choice. But in the background were other compelling decisions. The first was whether to join one of the fraternities on campus. Dad had done so at CSU, and, in the only brief conversation we had about college, he encouraged me to join the same fraternity. I am sure he thought this would be "good" for my social development. I joined, and though I have maintained life-long friendships, the results for social development were decidedly mixed. There were rituals I was not entirely comfortable with. Hell Week, billed as an experience to deeply bond fellow pledges, was truly out of the underworld's handbook.

I was also going to compete in varsity athletics, either wrestling or gymnastics. I decided to become a member of the gymnastics team. A factor in this decision was the influence of someone I knew through Don Robinson. Charles Jackson was on the high school team Don coached before assuming his position at ASU. Charles was also on the gymnastics team and a member of the same fraternity I pledged. He was of the highest character, somewhat in the mold of Don. As fraternity pledges, we selected pledge fathers. I was fortunate to be able to select him. Following graduation, he served in Vietnam as a decorated helicopter pilot.

In my senior year I was elected to an unsought leadership position, president of the Chapter with over 100 members. In contrast to most sororities and fraternities, the members were a heterogeneous lot, from truly rowdy partiers to serious scholar-athletes like Charles Jackson. It was the former which caused me trouble as president. I was once brought before the Assistant Dean of Students and bluntly informed that if I did not curtail the boisterous off-campus partying by some members, the university would. Again, my desire to shun controversy and avoid direct confrontation with the perpetrators was problematic, but, with no exit, I did as instructed.

Being president of a large fraternity resulted in my nomination to compete to be King, or some such Overlord, at a major intra-sorority function. I was told I would be brought before a group of sorority members to field questions as a part of the process. I had not considered the type of queries I might be asked nor prepared any answers, not even in a preliminary way, though I knew I was not good at "winging" it. I donned my red fraternity blazer and was shown into a room with more sorority members seated around the table than I had imagined would be there. The first question was something along the lines of, "what would it mean to you if you were to be selected?" I blathered a response as the color of my face began to approximate that of my blazer. It was downhill from there; I was not selected.

Tim also joined the fraternity I had pledged. He majored in electrical engineering, taking courses I could not fathom. Since we lived in the same fraternity house, my access to him was of immense help in courses like calculus and physics. In turn, I helped him in those courses wherein his dyslexia was most problematic. We had started this helpful pattern in high school, but this intensified in college. (As an aside, Tim achieved an A in every course within his major, and only one B in his remaining courses!). Though I passed calculus and other math courses with decent marks, largely thanks to Tim's help, physics was particularly hard, dominated as it was by so many equations. Later in life I began to read multiple authors, such as Frank Wilczek,[10] who have described the beauty of physics for an educated lay public in (mostly) equation-free prose.

School work was consuming as was gymnastics. I knew it would take a significant effort to close the competitive gap. I competed in only two events, floor exercise and trampoline (later removed from college gymnastics). I won meets on the trampoline during the first two years, but the competition was subpar. In my junior year a new coach, Stephen Johnson, was hired. He was the NCAA trampoline champion in 1962 and placed second at the World Professional Trampoline Championships in 1964. Over the years he remained coach he brought the program to a new level of respectability, and certainly improved my skills and placings. CSU seemed to have hired a notable talent. He became heavily involved in national and international gymnastics, staging numerous events involving Chinese and Russian teams.

Unfortunately, Stephen's life was to take a decidedly different turn than that of Don Robinson. Several years after I graduated from CSU, I was talking on the phone with my college advisor and friend, Dr. Robert Martin. He mentioned that at a recent meet, the gymnastics team refused to take the floor and compete for their coach. I never found out the reason(s) and did not ask. He was either fired or voluntarily left. I can only surmise this ambitious coach had taken on too many duties and was not devoting enough time to his CSU team? I was embarrassed for him from afar. This most promising coach, smart and talented, ultimately died in Nederland, Colorado at the age of 57.

When I made the switch to pre-med, I was assigned a new advisor, the aforementioned Dr. Martin, a professor of biochemistry. His field of expertise was steroid biochemistry. There are many classes of steroids which impact multiple bodily processes. After obtaining his PhD, Dr. Martin completed a Postdoctoral Fellowship at the University of Basel in Switzerland in the laboratory of Dr. Thaddeus Reichstein, a Nobel laureate who helped to isolate cortisone, a hormone secreted by the adrenal gland, and a compound which plays a central role in the body's response to stress. Dr. Martin's laboratory trained many scholars who subsequently had distinguished careers. His total commitment to his pre-med students was recognized when he received the Distinguished Service Award for Undergraduate Advising. Many students became his lifelong friends, and while at CSU were invited along on his frequent skiing, biking, and hiking trips.

In later years his mind, so attuned to science, the arts, and literature, became progressively dimmed by the scourge of Alzheimer's disease. He struggled mightily to maintain coherence and a connection with the wider world with which he had engaged so vibrantly. As he was entering the first phases of his disease, he began to send me his detailed musings on great scientists like Galileo and the science/religion interface as he interpreted it from his Unitarian Universalist background. I attended his last talk from the pulpit as a UU layperson. He was still lucid; his erudition ranged from astronomy to the evolution/creationism divide. As his mind clouded, he spent long hours on a paper he titled *A Search for the Historical Jesus*. Could he have picked a more difficult topic to research? I was gratified, however, that he sought my opinion on his many "treatises."

He had enlisted in the Army Air Corps in 1942 where he served as flight instructor and flew fighter planes between bases in the U.S. He had one harrowing flying experience due to inclement weather which he had told me about years before. The last time I called him, his disease was painfully evident. When the discussion flagged and he uttered "damn memory," he again launched into a rendition of this WWII story. It was evident this was one of the last memory traces to survive the ravages. This constriction of his conscious perception was frustrating for him and painful for his family and those close to him to observe. At his memorial service in the Unitarian Universalist church in Ft. Collins, many hundreds attended. The stories and fulsome praise for this man were an apt tribute and remembrance of him.

My third year in college I was introduced to a pert sorority member, an identical twin. Martha and I dated for about two years. In the final year both of us were presidents of our respective social houses, so we had that shared experience as a backdrop to voice our complaints. It was largely a chaste affair, though there was passion. Upon graduation I sort of melted away without much discussion of a future together. Many years later, after she divorced, she called and we resumed a friendship, warmed by our previous relationship. Over the years she has taught me many lessons about courage when confronting a myriad of life-threatening health problems. Her health history has also reinforced a lesson I have learned over many decades, the primacy of genetics in the causation of many disease states. Most diseases are due to a combination of predisposing genetic factors interacting with environmental influences. In her case, genetic factors predominated. She and her identical twin, with the same genes and same environment, developed the same serious diseases later in life, all within approximately the same time frame, one of which caused the death of her co-twin.

After the application and interview process for medical school admission, I elected to go to Baylor College of Medicine in Houston, Texas. Its reputation as a world-class cardiovascular center may have been the glitter, but the school had numerous strengths. Several of Dr. Martin's former advisees had attended this medical school, subsequently had successful careers, and reported positively to Dr. Martin about their experiences at Baylor. One of his advisees who attended this medical school, Lynn Loriaux, MD, PhD, became chairman of the department of Internal Medicine at the University of Oregon Medical School.

During my undergraduate years dad was living in Boulder, a short drive from Ft. Collins. Tim and I often went to Boulder and studied in the library on campus, always combined with a visit. Though we had this contact, dad and I never discussed in any depth my decision to enter medicine, a subject hived off from conversation. Though I did not consider it then, I would learn from events at Baylor that he sensed I was vulnerable to the depression he experienced when he entered medical school. If I perceived this correctly, this was no doubt a source of guilt and unease, a reason to stifle any conversation which would reveal our emotional relatedness.

Another source of tension for him seemed to be his continuing need to hide his sexual identity. He was never visited by another man when Tim and I came to Boulder. However, near the end of undergraduate school I had the sense, cobbled from small bits of observations, that he was gay. This produced a welter of emotions. The realization, of course, aided my understanding of my parents' separateness, though not in a salutary way. Yet over time I have developed compassion for his circumstance. It made sense that he would closet his sexual orientation. The wider world, at that time, considered his homosexuality a product of broken, debauched humanity. As I graduated college I was bewildered and conflicted, though curious about this utterly alien life. I was drawn to persons and ideas on the margin.

⁛

I ENROLLED at Baylor College of Medicine in 1966. The history of this school was dominated by two central figures, Dr. Michael DeBakey, the feisty son of a Lebanese merchant family that had immigrated to Lake Charles, Louisiana, and Dr. Denton Cooley, a tall, low-key, native Texan son of a dentist. Though both were cardiovascular surgeons and peers, Dr.

Cooley became Dr. DeBakey's de facto protégé after the heart-lung machine was developed in 1955 and open-heart surgery became possible. They operated together, published papers, and developed and perfected techniques. The clear boss, however, was Dr. DeBakey. Dr. Cooley, chafing under this relationship, moved from Methodist Hospital to St. Luke's, still connected with the medical school, and established the Texas Heart Institute.

Key developments intersected this history, including the first heart transplant performed in South Africa by Dr. Christiaan Barnard in 1967. Surgeons in several major centers in the U.S. followed suite, including Drs. Cooley and DeBakey. There was an area above Dr. BeBakey's operating room where medical students, physicians at various stages of training, and visiting physicians could crane over a railing encircling a glassed-in portion of the ceiling and view procedures. When DeBakey was going to perform a heart transplant, news would sweep through campus and fellow students, assuming it was not class time, would dash to Methodist Hospital to secure a favorable position at the railing.

Dr. Cooley had developed considerable expertise operating on infants and children with congenital (born with) heart defects. His technical skill and speed were legendary. I rotated through his service as part of a surgical clerkship and scrubbed in as observer on several cases. His demeanor was calm, his voice never raised. On rounds at the end of the day, his entry into a room was met with reverence by the family. His good looks and earnestness were captivating.

Dr. DeBakey's personality contrasted sharply. As Chancellor of the medical school, he sat atop a structured hierarchy and was infamous for terrorizing those beneath. His surgical training program included a full month on his service for every surgical intern, no time off, mostly taking care of his often very ill postoperative patients and assuring those admitted for surgery had the proper work-up. A friend who had endured this month described the bone-deep fatigue and the fear lest DeBakey find fault. Some surgical interns did not make it through this sieve.

The rift between Drs. Cooley and DeBakey deepened when Dr. DeBakey accused Dr. Cooley of "stealing" ideas related to DeBakey's cherished goal of an artificial heart and lured one of DeBakey's key aides to join the Cooley team. This history has been well documented.[11] Their storied relationship entered the national press and popular imagination with the publication of a 1970 *Life* magazine featuring a picture of the two men on the cover with the caption *A Bitter Feud: Two Great Surgeons at War Over the Human Heart.*

A less publicized rift also involved two titans of science, taking place at Baylor over many years.[12] Competition among scientists can be bare-knuckled. This one was particularly rife with conflict, involving Andrew Schally and Roger Guillemin, investigators in the nascent field of brain hormone research, specifically releasing factors in the hypothalamus that stimulate the release of hormones from the pituitary gland. In the early years of their ego-driven competition they attempted to isolate and chemically characterize corticotropin releasing factor (CRF), the molecule which begins the key pathway of the stress response. CRF causes the pituitary to synthesize and release the hormone ACTH which, in turn, is the signal for the adrenal gland to release cortisol. As previously noted, my college advisor, Dr. Robert Martin, completed Fellowship training in the laboratory of the scientist who isolated cortisol, Dr. Thaddeus Reichstein, earning his advisor the Nobel Prize. In 1977 Drs. Schally and Guillemin garnered the Nobel Prize for their work in this fascinating field.

This was the backdrop for me and the other students, 80 males and two females, in my class. It was a demanding environment, though most of the intriguing details about these clashes in the clinical realm and in the laboratory remained in the background as we immersed ourselves in the grind of lectures, laboratories, and book work. Perhaps a holdover from the previous ties to the undergraduate (Baptist) campus in Waco (which Dr. DeBakey had severed), the Dean of Students, without specific mention, expected probity, reflected in the requirement that males wear ties to class lectures. A significant minority of the students came from Ivy League schools. Not unexpectedly, the atmosphere was competitive, and the volume of material could quickly become overwhelming.

I was not alone in feeling inundated. Soon after first-year classes began, we were seated in front of microscopes in histology class in alphabetical order. Thus, I sat next to Stuart Yudofsky, an undergraduate English major from New York. He had an artist's sensibility, and though he passed the required courses to enter medical school, his thought patterns gravitated toward the literary. When first staring down the tube of a microscope to view a section of liver, he was clearly flummoxed, and implored me to tell him what, exactly, he was looking at. We bonded over these experiences.

He was a writer and poet; he continued to write poetry while in medical school. I considered some of the poems to be achievements of the highest order. He became a long-term Chair of the Department of Psychiatry at Baylor College of Medicine and author or co-author of many papers and books. His English background had served him well.

Students were encouraged to attend lectures given by scientists from other institutions. Baylor, a school with robust research in many areas, exemplified by the work of Nobel laureates cited earlier, was frequently visited by notable scholars. There seemed to be heightened interest when it was announced that Jacques Monod, a Nobel Prize winner in 1965, would be giving a talk on work he and others had conducted which led to this coveted award. An aura surrounded this man. Monod had become friends with Albert Camus when both joined the French underground resistance in WWII.[13] This elegant Frenchman drew a large crowd, primarily because the research was the first demonstration that genes are turned "on" and "off."[14] The work, conducted in the bacterium *Escherichia coli* (*E. coli*)—but applicable to all of life's Kingdoms—revealed a fundamental mechanism by which genes are regulated, pointing the way to an understanding of how the genes of an organism orchestrate development, metabolism, and a host of other functions.

E. coli can survive and grow rapidly when fed either glucose (their preferred food source) or lactose. Monod and François Jacob discovered that when both sugars are present, the growth is rapid, followed by a short pause, then by a return to rapid growth. These men showed that glucose metabolizing proteins were present during the first phase of growth, then wane as the glucose supply is exhausted, followed by resumption of growth as lactose metabolizing proteins appear. The genes responsible for glucose utilization are turned "on" (activated), then "off" (repressed), succeeded in turn by activation of lactose metabolizing genes as lactose is consumed. It is as if the cells "know" when gene products are needed and when not. This work was one of the most significant signposts which began the "molecular revolution." The atmosphere in the room was electric. Though I did not understand much of the talk, I sensed the beauty, the satisfaction of designing and carrying out experiments which explain many disparate observations. Science, in this sense, can serve as an anchor, an enterprise that can be trusted. In this process the truths of the natural world are ferreted out. Facts are built upon facts, creating a sturdy edifice.

In addition to course work, freshmen students were expected to conduct a mentored research project and present the results to the mentor's department. A fortunate happenstance, born of necessity, played a role in my selection of a project and favorably influenced future decisions and opportunities. The Chair of the Department of Anatomy, Dr. Robert Liebelt, MD, PhD, was a short man with a fringe of hair rimming his large head which seemed to merge directly with his shoulders. His cherubic countenance was matched by an open, welcoming disposition. I was in a position faced by many students, scrambling to pay for this education. As I was walking the hallway early in my first year, I passed his office. He was seated at his desk, and, upon impulse, I walked in through the open doorway. His friendly greeting allowed me to ask if he had any duties in the department which would provide some remuneration. He puzzled the question, and, after a pause during which I felt I may have intruded, he indicated he had given a small space to an engineer, not on the faculty, to test some of his theories about high pressure, analogous to the increasing pressure as a diver descends into a body of water. In his spare time this engineer had published on pressure effects on biological systems in a theoretical journal.[15] It was typical of Dr. Liebelt to support a fringe scientist whose work he found intriguing. He introduced me to the engineer, Mr. Karl Doerner, in his borrowed room containing small steel chambers he had designed and built, with pass-through attachments to tanks of gas; oxygen, nitrogen, and helium.

Mr. Doerner was self-funding his research. He was tall with a scraggly beard; over time I came to appreciate his eccentricity. Dr. Liebelt explained that I would be available on weekends to compress mice to a predetermined "depth" and, usually a day later, decompress these mice housed in the chambers. For the pressure profiles we had to calculate the percentage of the mixed gas ingredients, progressively decreasing oxygen and nitrogen during the compression phase (with helium added for the higher pressures) and reversing the process upon decompression. The titration of the gases was critical. Too much oxygen at a given pressure causes brain and lung damage, too little had the consequences we are all familiar with. Also to be avoided was decompression sickness, the release of nitrogen dissolved in the tissues in excess of that which can be safely eliminated by respiration. The decompression profile had to avoid nitrogen bubbles in the tissues, the cause of this malady. Thus, the gas mixture had to be adjusted during the many hours' long decompression. After I learned the system, I devised some straightforward experiments I could parlay into my freshman research project. This met with Mr. Doerner's approval, since it was clear he had not devised experiments which could bridge the gap between his theoretical models of pressure effects on cells and those on biological systems of intact animals. This was my first of many future research projects which would involve mice.

Dr. Liebelt's department maintained a large colony of inbred strains of mice, some with predispositions to diseases such as diabetes, obesity, and other conditions. Though there were other facilities in the country devoted to mouse research, such as the Jackson Laboratory in Bar Harbor, Maine, Dr. Liebelt was prescient in his recognition of the value such a facility would have for his faculty and other investigators on campus. Dr. Liebelt, ever curious in an almost childlike way, performed research on mice well into his 80s.

As the first year of medical school proceeded and the work, within and outside the formal curriculum, became unrelenting, I began to experience increasing feelings of profound unease and dysphoria. It took me some time to put labels to these symptoms of depression and anxiety. Precursors to these states were present much earlier in life, but now they were starkly felt, so much so they seemed alien. These two demons are often linked. Genetic predisposition becomes exposed to myriad, swirling environmental factors, setting the conditions for these disorders to manifest. It is beyond dispute that anxiety and depression are highly heritable and become unmasked or exacerbated by a stress-inducing environment. To state these truths again, so many of the diseases physicians encounter in practice, including depression and anxiety, are multifactorial, resulting from a bewildering combination of the genes one is born with (innate factors) and the surroundings one encounters within the larger environment.

I was unprepared for this onslaught, as anyone is. Along with so many distressing symptoms and feeling states, perhaps the most troubling, and the one inflaming all others, was the sleep disturbance. I did not sleep well before, but the quality and quantity of sleep deteriorated further, and there was no time during the day to get rest. To adequately describe any of this is beyond my poor abilities. Though these feeling states are difficult for anyone to accurately describe, many writers have been eloquent on the subject. One author whose descriptions sound true is William Styron.[16] At various points in his short "memoir of madness" he writes: "Depression is a disorder of mood, so mysteriously painful and elusive in the way it becomes known to the self—to the mediating intellect—as to verge close to being beyond description. It thus remains nearly incomprehensible to those who have not experienced it in its extreme mode. ... gloom crowding in on me, a sense of dread and alienation, and, above all, stifling anxiety.... My brain had begun to endure its familiar siege: panic and dislocation, and a sense that my thought processes were being engulfed by a toxic and unnameable tide that obliterated any enjoyable response to the living world. ... The disruption of normal sleep patterns is a notoriously devastating feature of depression. ... Although as an illness depression manifests certain unvarying characteristics, it also allows for many idiosyncrasies; I've been amazed at some of the freakish phenomena—not reported by other patients—that it has wrought amid the twistings of my mind's labyrinth. ... Never let it be doubted that depression, in its extreme form, is madness. The madness results from an aberrant biochemical process. It has been established with reasonable certainty (after strong resistance from many psychiatrists, and not all that long ago) that such madness is chemically induced amid the neurotransmitters of the brain, probably as the result of systemic stress, which for unknown reasons causes depletion of the chemicals norepinephrine and serotonin, and the increase of a hormone, cortisol. With all this upheaval in the brain tissues, the alternate drenching and deprivation, it is no wonder that the mind begins to feel aggrieved, stricken, and the muddied thought processes register the distress of an organ in convulsion."

The general observations quoted above were true to my experience. It was daily and unrelenting. It may be thought that I overdramatize or exaggerate. I can only report my lived experience. I did not, however, seriously consider leaving school. The one firm template I had for getting through was wrestling; keep moving, don't, metaphorically speaking, lie down in the snow and give up. I did not consciously bring wrestling to mind in the service of placing one foot ahead of the other, showing up every day, but the approach required the same turn of mind.

Toward the end of the first year, an unusual confluence led to the potential for help, though this proved not to be the case. A faculty member in biochemistry at Baylor knew my college advisor, Dr. Robert Martin, and invited him to give one of our lectures. Dr. Martin, who I have indicated was such a positive influence as my pre-med advisor in undergraduate school, had met my father in the past and called him to ask if he had any messages he would like him, Dr. Martin, to convey to me when he came to Houston. Perhaps thinking back to his reaction the first time he enrolled in medical school, he asked Dr. Martin to arrange psychological help if he thought it was warranted. There had been no communication between dad and me, so this request had to have been based on little more than intuition. Today I think about the scene in the bedroom in Rye, him in obvious emotional distress, his hand on my thigh, both staring at the ceiling, both of us locked in a tortured silence. It was as if he knew I would share his misery when confronted by similar circumstances and was communicating this awful fate to my young self.

Dr. Martin gently inquired about my well-being and told me about his conversation with dad. I said just enough to convince him. Dr. Martin was always one to cut through niceties and impediments. He made an appointment that day with a senior member of the department of psychiatry. I went to his office the next day and, after the briefest of conversations, he recommended psychoanalysis (yes, psychoanalysis!). In high school I had taken a horseback trip on mountain trails, organized by an outfitting group. On this trip I met a lawyer from the east coast who had undergone intensive analysis (many years, five days a week). He was forthcoming about this experience; for unclear reasons he wanted to communicate how this intense process had helped him. Was he sensing something I was projecting? While sharing this with me he seemed the most together, intelligent person I had met to that date. I, therefore, had a sense of what was required, was intellectually drawn to this exotic method of probing the mind, and thought it could help. It did not take long for me to discern there was probably not another form of therapy I was less equipped to benefit from.

I was paired with a taciturn, slightly obese man with a crew cut. Even at the first session he said little more than that the sessions required I be prone on the couch and utter whatever came to my mind, free association. It was customary that five sessions per week were required, but I would be "allowed" the minimum of three. The rate would be reduced because I was a student, and I would be billed even if I missed a session. Students were not afforded medical insurance at that time. The therapist sat in a chair at the head of the couch overlooking my outstretched frame. He lit a cigarette, then one after the other. Before the session ended, I had mumbled a few sentences. Thus began a year I am embarrassed to relate.

Dr. Sigmund Freud developed free association as the mechanism to uncover deep psychic wounds and produce insights. The patient was to speak anything which came to mind, a stream of consciousness, including dreams or fragments of dreams, as the path to access the unconscious. This was so far beyond any mental tool I might be able to bring to the therapeutic setting (particularly with this physician) as to be utterly unavailable to me. (Though dad was talkative, he was largely absent. I did not grow up in a verbal household, a state I contributed to. I was closed, sharing almost nothing with emotional content either inside or outside the home). My verbalizations on the couch were infrequent and inchoate. Portnoy I was not! Despite what I tried to convince myself was a good faith effort (though, of course, it wasn't), these sessions often went by with only a few words from me and none from him, aside from an occasional "uhm." His chain smoking and occasional release of intestinal gas was the pall through which I was to offer up snippets of material, harvested deep inside the mind, to ultimately weave a tale that would unshackle the past and provide a new way of being. Yes, I will concede I was "resistant," a term much in vogue when the process fails. As I view these sessions from a remove of many decades, it strikes me this qualifies as theater of the absurd, hour upon hour of a near-static frame whirring by. I was having significant difficulty during this and subsequent periods of life. Perhaps I squandered an opportunity, but after a year I did not see a glimmer of hope I would get better through this process and ended analysis with a profound sense of failure.

At several times during this year of analysis I remember a feeling that things/existence were/was not "real;" a distinct sense of unreality; brief episodes, but stunning and deeply distressing when they occurred. By this I do not mean unreality in the way schizophrenic patients experience unreality. I thought by bringing it up in a session, this might be an opening for a wider exploration. When I related that I had this fleeting sense that things were not real, his response was a dismissive "Oh sure," quashing any further discussion. It was as if he was derisively saying *where did you read that one*?

This stark sense of unreality, the experience of it from that period, has stayed with me and sparked readings on what constitutes bedrock reality. In the last chapter, I offer my synthesis of reality, co-mingled with a psychiatric perspective and an admixture of consciousness.

To pay for analysis and school, I had many different jobs throughout, most of them hospital based. Two opportunities provided the greatest financial help. Toward the end of the first year, Dr. Liebelt inquired if I might want to consider splitting the second-year classes, and in the process obtain a Master's (MS) degree in his department in addition to the MD degree, though it would take an extra year. This opportunity, which would provide some federal funding for two years, was open to five students in the first-year class. I applied and was selected. One of our five members was Peter Kennedy who attended Harvard undergraduate school and subsequently became the class Valedictorian. Whereas learning could be drudgery for most of us, he absolutely loved learning. He became an oncologist, a fitting specialty for him. Each cancer is a different disease. The myriad types and the knowledge to be learned about each no doubt has satisfied his urge to know.

Our responsibilities as "split-year" students were to help teach in the gross anatomy (with cadavers) and neuroanatomy labs for first year students, as well as in histology. Neuroanatomy was a singular experience: holding slices of someone's brain in the palm of my hand, surveying the infolding surface of the cerebral cortex, grey matter, the underlying white matter through which messages are conveyed over myelin-ensheathed cables, the deeper nuclei of grey matter which participate in the neural relays, the brainstem housing nuclei which control functions which require no conscious consideration such as breathing, the hindmost cerebellum which in life controls movement, but also houses cognitive functions, all of these structures supporting the immensely complex life of the generous donor of this brain.

We also took graduate level classes, taught mostly to students obtaining MS and PhD degrees, and we were expected to perform and write a thesis to satisfy the MS requirements. This decision to pursue the extra year coincided with the decision to undergo analysis. With this split-year I was able to structure my time to accommodate these sessions. The choice of a project for the MS degree was to be a continuation of work with mice, utilizing the hyperbaric chambers.

The second opportunity was quite stressful, though it provided room and board; a Spartan room in a low, one-story cinderblock building without air conditioning on the VA hospital grounds, and food from the hospital cafeteria. There were different jobs available to students seeking this aid. Mine, after only two training sessions a couple of hours each, was to be the surgical scrub nurse, handing instruments to the surgeons performing emergency operations any time during the nights I was assigned. Usually everyone in the room was tired, even exhausted during these cases. It is common knowledge that surgeons, as a group, can be temperamental, even irascible. When the wrong instrument is given them, the needle not threaded quickly, or delay in passing instruments generally, this could raise the ire of the surgeon. But I have to say most were patient; I recall only one particularly irritated surgeon who did not address me personally but did growl unpleasantly into an open abdomen. I confess this rattled me considerably. I learned quickly and within a short time became proficient.

Though Dr. Liebelt was my thesis advisor, he was not knowledgeable, nor would he be expected to be, about an organism's adaptation, its physiology, when placed at higher pressures and decompressed. I was on my own, devising and carrying out the experiments. The basic finding when I did blood work, evaluated the organs under a microscope, and other studies was that these animals were stressed, the higher the pressure with its longer period of decompression, the greater the level of stress.

That these mice were being stressed should not have been a surprise, but at the time I had no knowledge of the vast literature related to stress from the time Hans Selye described a common response to stress as a syndrome, or collection of findings.[17] So much has subsequently been learned about stress as a central driving force in individual lives and, indeed, in its role promoting organismal adaptations in the struggle for existence. It was also no surprise that the stress response resonated with me and motivated a desire not only to understand what I was seeing with the mice, but to understand stress within its broader context in the energy, economy, and emotional vicissitudes of life. This desire has not abated. I wrote up the thesis, which was approved by my thesis committee, before I started the final two years of medical school in the clinics and on the hospital wards, and, occasionally in the operating rooms.

As Dr. Liebelt entered his eighth decade we began communicating again, and I visited him once at his residence in Ohio. His life had taken many interesting turns. The year I graduated, 1971, he left Baylor to become the first Provost at the Medical College of Georgia. Three years later he helped start a new medical school in Ohio, becoming Provost and charter Dean of the Northeast Ohio Universities College of Medicine. In 1982 he shifted his life's work completely to become director of Addiction Medicine at St. Thomas Hospital in Akron, the first hospital in the country to have an entire ward dedicated to the treatment of alcoholics. When I visited him in his later 80s, he gave me a CD of the lecture he personally gave his patients. It was vintage Dr. Liebelt, Sharpie in hand, arrows going in all directions on the whiteboard, explaining the way alcohol is metabolized and the damage thereby inflicted. By the end, almost every square inch of the whiteboard was covered. These sessions were attended not only by the patients on the ward, but often by their relatives and other interested parties. Though unconventional, his patients responded to this direct teaching and caring attitude. By his admittedly imprecise statistics, Dr. Liebelt's rate of relapse was low.

The lectures he provided on this ward were reminiscent of the well-received lectures he gave to medical students, using colored chalk and the blackboard. As an aside, he may have been influenced by an older German anatomist in his department at Baylor, Dr. Arnold Zimmerman, schooled during an era when learning was more formal. He was our lecturer for the head and neck portion of the anatomy class. He came to class with five colors of chalk, white (bone), red (artery), blue (vein), brown (muscle), and yellow (nerve). For tendons, he skillfully merged the brown of muscle into the white of tendon. He also brought a bucket of water and rag. He would begin a large drawing, perfectly placed, expounding in his thick German accent as he continued the drawing. The anatomy emerged almost life-like from the black background; chalk dust enveloped the space around him, his white lab coat a pastiche of these colors. We thought of each of these drawings, class after class, as masterpieces. They could have been framed and placed in a gallery or used in a textbook. At the conclusion of each he dipped his rag into the bucket and swiftly wiped away these treasures.

Dr. Liebelt continued to see patients until age 80. The locals who revered him called him "Dr. Bob." As a "habit" he could not shed, he maintained a mouse colony and, believing that bee pollen has health benefits, he began to evaluate the health consequences of feeding mice only bee pollen granules and water. These mice did surprisingly well.[18] As he approached age 90 the results of these experiments, which he essentially did on his own time, were self-published.[19]

With no benefit from psychoanalysis, my depression/anxiety continued. There was no talk of medication during this year of therapy, nor with analysis being "talk" therapy would one expect such a recommendation. The available medications were less efficacious than those available today and have more side effects. Over the years I have returned to a therapist's office, each for a variable length of time, with variable degrees of helpfulness. These professionals have urged medication in addition to talk therapy; the combination is more efficacious than either form of treatment alone.[20] I have tried numerous medications. I am among those for whom the drugs (at least those I was prescribed) either did not work or had significant side effects. One outcome over the recent several years in therapy has been the growing conviction that the optimal means to tell the science I wish to convey is via a personal narrative as background in the service of this goal. It is clear to me I would not be able to pen these highly personal details in the absence of ongoing therapy, though doing so remains an uncomfortable task.

Enduring the daily medical school grind and meeting others' expectations (I was certainly not meeting mine) was about the extent of what I could manage. Expending the energy to socialize, find a date and then muster the resources to actually be in that person's company in a companionable way, was a goal I would pursue in the future. However, this posture was not to last. At some point during my third year an acquaintance was breaking up with a woman he had been dating, and, perhaps out of guilt, wondered if I might want to meet her. She worked as a laboratory technician in the "charity" hospital, Ben Taub. I knew she was attractive, but little more than that. My time with her precipitated a decision with long-lasting consequences.

After several dates, wherein she carried most of the conversational load and thus spared me, it was evident sexual relations were to follow. I did like her, and with sexual activity deferred for such a long time, I was an eager participant. I did not ask, nor did she offer, any information about birth control. Reluctant to broach the subject, I assumed she must be on birth control. Within a short period of time after we met, she informed me she was pregnant. Nothing was said for an interminable period. I was in total despair. I did not know the experience of love but was certain I did not love her and was in no position financially or emotionally to have a baby. She, for her part, pushed for an agreement that if she consented to an abortion, we would later marry. I did not agree to this. Several days later she said she would have an abortion.

What to do? This was pre-Roe v. Wade. I made an appointment with a physician I had met in the course of one of my jobs. I sensed I could broach this difficult subject. He proved to be sensitive and he knew the options. It seemed I was not the first student who had faced this wrenching decision. He gave me the phone number and address of someone who, he said, performed safe abortions. When I drove to his large, isolated mansion at night with cash in hand, it was evident he garnered a sizeable income. I am ashamed to this day I was thinking only about myself and, at least during those initial stages, not about the life which had been created. In the months following I had the awful sense I was a murderer, and in some sense of that word I was. This feeling would sweep over me in a manner reminiscent of that occasioned by the fleeting sense of unreality. I did not share this with my companion. She said little about the abortion, and in short order seemed back to her baseline, though she may have been concealing grief I did not or could not discern.

Years later I chose subspecialty training in Medical Genetics following an Ob/Gyn residency. This has translated to decades of counseling women and couples faced with the abortion decision when one of the prenatal tests and/or an ultrasonogram had revealed the fetus she was carrying had an abnormality or collection of abnormalities of varying degrees of severity. Though their decisions came under circumstances vastly different from mine, I felt I had some insight into the swirling, complex emotions which accompany this decision. I hear from patients years after they have either made the decision to terminate or carry the affected pregnancy. In general, they are grateful they were presented their options in a non-directive manner. I have always been struck by the persisting impact of these decisions years, even decades, later.

In the middle of this turmoil, with a few days off, I made the impulsive decision to drive to visit dad, now residing in Denver. I don't know the motivation, though am sure it was to attempt some mutual understanding, forge some alliance to buffer the anguish. If we were locked in the same battles, then perhaps talking about it, as had never been done, might help.

I called to ask if I could come for a visit. There was hesitation, but he said yes, seeming distant. In short order after I arrived it became evident the timing was darkly inauspicious. He was despondent. Perhaps he thought he could conceal this for a day or two. He could not. A relationship with an Ob/Gyn physician had ended, and he was frankly suicidal. Our roles quickly reversed, though I would not be able to handle the situation for long. I called my good brother, now pursuing MD *and* PhD degrees at the University of Washington. Tim flew to Denver and took dad to Seattle. I got in the car and drove back to Houston; a longer trip I have never experienced.

Tim recognized that dad was suicidal, but he resisted hospitalization. Tim, therefore, sought a court order for commitment which a judge granted. Dad was hospitalized at the VA in Seattle. The initial recommendation was electroconvulsive therapy. During one of his prior episodes of depression he had undergone this form of treatment, which caused memory loss for a time and was very troubling to him. Though electroconvulsive therapy had fewer such side effects at the time of his Seattle hospitalization, he declined this recommendation, but did allow a trial of medications. After a month he had improved sufficiently to be discharged. Tim had seen him through a dangerous period.

I entered the final two years of clinical work unsure about a career choice. We had rotations on the various specialty services which would allow a student to decide. The last rotation my final year was Ob/Gyn at the Jefferson Davis hospital where, at that time, approximately 10,000 babies were born each year. Students were pressed into duty. It was literally observe a delivery, perform one with a senior resident supervising, and then the student, assuming he or she did the delivery well, performed unaided deliveries of women who had already had at least one infant, had an uncomplicated pregnancy, with the infant-to-be presenting head-first. It was not unsafe. The nurse in the delivery room was a savvy observer, and knew when things were not going well, in which case she would quickly fetch a resident to the room. I enjoyed Ob/Gyn and would likely have applied for training in this field had this rotation come earlier, but a decision about further training was required prior to my Ob/Gyn rotation. Unsure about the "right" course, I applied for a pediatric internship in the Baylor program when the time came to do so.

Depression/anxiety continued as constant companions during the clinical years, to be joined by that malign spike of pernicious neural activity I had first experienced when rolled up in mats in high school, trying to sweat off a few ounces to make weight for the upcoming wrestling match. I refer to panic. It did not happen often. To someone who has not experienced panic, I cannot possibly describe the sheer terror which is this singular experience, manufactured by temporarily disordered neural pathways and their associated chemicals. It arises unbidden, begins with dread, though with no "real" external threat, only the internal turmoil which is scrambled and reinterpreted in the brain of the afflicted person. In its textbook presentation, a person in the throes of a full-blown attack (as opposed to "panicky" feelings) has multiple physical symptoms (racing heart, difficulty breathing), coupled with bizarre mental symptoms, often producing a feeling one is "going crazy" or is having a heart attack and may die. This malady demonstrates the tight association between the mental (brain) and the rest of the physical body, both displaying prominent symptoms of panic. These symptoms manifest as the dread builds, and, at its peak, consciousness is constricted, squeezed to a peephole and then any semblance of usual consciousness is relinquished, giving way to overwhelming feelings of anxiety and frantic agitation. Reason and logical thinking are precluded.

Panic sets off a train of counterregulatory measures, a fevered attempt to reassert some semblance of equilibrium. How this is accomplished no one knows. If we knew this—and what precipitates these attacks/states—we would know a treasure trove of neuroscience. After "recovery" from one of these episodes, I sat down and dropped into an oddly reflective state. In that moment, inexplicably, I was awed by this experience and became curious about what had transpired at the neural circuit and cellular/molecular levels. It became at once intensely frightening but also intensely interesting.

If this is read—and it would be OK if it was only Marilyn, Tim, and a few friends—the reader would be justified to be skeptical. I have not told anyone about the extra-school struggles except a mention or two to Tim and, later, a medical faculty colleague. How does one continue? Contemporary accounts of severe depression[21] and anxiety,[22] written from a first-person perspective, show that one can live with extremes of these disorders and still function, though this usually requires medication. Persons with other debilitating handicaps prevail against all odds. Tim, with severe dyslexia, obtained MD and PhD degrees in addition to a BS in electrical engineering.

People compensate and persevere, optimizing their strengths as a hedge against their frailties.

Also, I know that among my classmates I was not alone. Complicating everyone's life at that time was the general unrest in the nation; the Vietnam War and the protests, drugs, and a host of other social ills. Because I opted for the split-year program, I knew students from two classes, about 165. Of this group, followed into their training or beginning years of practice, two had committed suicide, one died of a drug overdose, and two died of AIDS.

⁝⁝⁝

I DID GRADUATE. My good sister came to the ceremony. Then I began to prepare for an internship. This year was as arduous as advertised. My first month was spent in the Emergency Room in the Ben Taub hospital, seeing all comers, not just the children. The volume we cared for was overwhelming. Most of the city's major trauma cases (shootings, stabbings, car wrecks, etc.) came here. When, for instance, a shooting victim was brought to the ER, all interns and residents were to come to that room and lend assistance. In the meantime, all the other patients you were responsible for continued to flood in, and in short order one could fall pitiably behind. Given the volume and severity of the cases and frenetic pace, I often imagined the contents of this war zone would just spill out into the streets.

Being so busy and stressed in entirely novel ways with this raft of responsibilities seemed to shift the inner-generated depression/anxiety into different channels; not easier, just different. The sheer magnitude of suffering we witnessed, the amount of work demanded, and the required attention fostered a more other-directed approach. It was mandatory that one brought focus and concentration to this work to provide effective (and safe) care. I even now reminisce about the ward where so many of the children with acute lymphocytic leukemia were treated. The mortality rate for this disease at that time was quite high. I vividly recall the struggles of the children and their parents. Fortunately, in a few short decades this rate has reversed; most affected children are now survivors. Medicine has advanced on many fronts, but this is one of the most gratifying stories from my perspective.

This focus and concentration were temporarily sidelined when I received a call from Marie Bell, dad's office nurse in Rifle and merciful tutor when I was having trouble in grade school, with news dad could not personally tell me. He had hit a six-year-old child who had darted into the street between two cars. The accident was fatal. Years later when I was involved in a case which resulted in a fetal death following a high-risk intrauterine procedure, I felt culpable. I knew dad well enough to know he also felt culpable. These events were another link in our shared psyches stamped by genes and environment. There were likely few days he was spared thoughts of that event. Striking and killing a child and feeling responsible for a fetal death are stark examples of the jumble of negative intrusive thoughts which can assail the stream of consciousness; they are difficult to eradicate.

Recently my sister and I were going through a trunk of dad's personal effects, a chore we had put off for many years. In this seemingly random collection was a letter from my brother to dad, a kind, deeply felt message to assuage his guilt and let him know that he was loved by his youngest son and was admired for his courage when he was hospitalized in Seattle for psychiatric care. I had considered at the time of the accident I should call to offer solace or at least send a note—I was saddened this had happened—but this was overridden by conflicting currents of emotion.

One other item in the trunk was a lengthy piece of research he had typed titled *Geography of Mankind*. It dealt with overpopulation, land use, resources, cultural influences, and related subjects. I do not know what prompted him to undertake this scholarship but found it comforting that he evinced this level of concern for humankind. In my interactions with him he displayed a near constant self-referential focus.

As the internship was coming to an end, I had reached another decision point. I was unsure if I wanted to pursue pediatrics as a career. I considered the options, including military service. The compulsory physician draft ended as the Vietnam War was winding down. I knew there were Navy facilities devoted to diving research and hyperbaric medicine (treating patients with certain conditions, such as burns, in a chamber with elevated levels of oxygen). I decided I would join the Navy, but only if I could fill an opening at such a facility. I sent my MS thesis dealing with hyperbaric physiology to the Bureau of Medicine and Surgery and explained my desire. Within a short time I heard back that, yes, I would be assigned to such a facility. To my dismay, the orders I ultimately received would have sent me to a Seabee unit in Shreveport, Louisiana as a General Medical Officer. There I would have taken care of these men and their family members after only a pediatric internship. Seabees were the builders in the Navy, including underwater construction. Perhaps this latter activity caused confusion and resulted in the orders I received.

At this point I did not know what else I was going to do. I felt trapped and became resigned to this fate. It would be two years and then I could get out. I discussed this dilemma with a physician friend who had been in the Navy. He advised I write my congressmen and explain what had happened. I was reluctant to do this, but I ultimately sat at the typewriter and wrote these letters. I included the letter from the Navy which had assured me a billet related to my research at Baylor. To my great relief I received an assignment to the Diving Research/Hyperbaric Medicine Branch of the Medical Research Facility at the Submarine Base in Groton, Connecticut.

⋄⋄⋄

THE FACILITY I joined, the Naval Submarine Medical Research Laboratory in Groton, Connecticut, was embedded within the larger submarine base across the Thames River from General Dynamics Electric Boat where these seagoing marvels of technology are built. The laboratory employed enlisted and civilian scientists from diverse fields, ranging from psychology and neuroscience to basic physiology. An older physician, Karl Schaeffer, was an expert on the physiologic effects of carbon dioxide, a small fraction of the atmosphere with adverse consequences for human well-being if elevated in either a diving or submarine setting. His first view of America was through the periscope of a German U-boat. I joined an ample scientific staff, sufficiently deep to conduct their individual research programs *and* contribute to a team approach on larger projects, as will be described.

Shortly after arriving I was given the option to participate in an intensive, month-long diving course at the Naval Shipyard on the Potomac River in Washington, D.C. I elected to attend as one of 12 physicians across the country involved with naval diving activities. The days were long and challenging; an early morning run followed by other exercises, class work on the basic principles of diving, written exams we had to pass, and "diving." The latter consisted of an imaginative combination of diving gear and locations. Hard helmets, rubber suits, and heavy boots were sometimes worn in a chamber partially filled with water; other dives with the same equipment were conducted while standing on a platform in a body of water near the Dahlgren,

Virginia Naval Base on a helium-oxygen mixture, pressurized in the suite to the depth-equivalent of 300 feet of sea water. Dives in dark, constricted spaces sometimes caused extreme discomfort, but successfully completing them provided a measure of confidence.

The Potomac River was the venue for the most unpleasant diving, which involved a device called a Jack Browne rig, basically a face mask covering eyes, nose, and mouth with connection to a surface hose supplying air and an attached valve controlling air flow into the mask. When it was my turn, I descended into what was, at that time, highly polluted water with swim trunks, fins, and the aforementioned breathing system. No light penetrated within a few feet of the surface. On the bottom, as I moved around, the airflow abruptly stopped. A rising sense of anxiety was tamped down when I remembered I could give three sharp tugs on the air hose, and I would be brought to the surface. Before resorting to this measure, I reached up and turned the valve, restoring airflow. I surmise the air hose had swept across the relatively loose valve, shutting it off. Because our ears were exposed to a truly polluted river, painful infections in the outer ear canals occurred in several classmates. Within a year the Navy Diving School was relocated to Panama City, Florida with its relatively pristine offshore waters.

Back at the base, I began talking in earnest with George Adams about experiments he had planned and had mentioned to me in a preliminary way before I left for diving school. George had a wide-ranging background, including chemistry and law degrees. He was a bold thinker, pressing his agenda in a manner which frequently rankled some of the more conservative members of the Navy brass. He was largely self-taught in the myriad aspects of diving, but able to mold a team with the expertise he lacked. Based on earlier work, he envisioned ways to increase the efficiency and lower the costs of underwater operations along a significant portion of the continental shelf. These operations could include salvage work and mineral and oil exploration (recall that it was the U.S. Navy initially overseeing the feasibility of oil extraction from shale rock around Rifle). The stated goals might be accomplished by placing working divers for an extended period in a chamber on air, submerged in seawater at a relatively shallow depth (50 to 60-foot seawater equivalent). Deeper dives or excursions to a work site on the ocean floor, again breathing air, could be undertaken, with return to the habitat without need for decompression. A relatively long period of decompression would be required when ascending to sea level, as the tissues would be fully saturated with nitrogen after the prolonged residence at 50 to 60 feet. The greater efficiency and cost savings could be substantial when weighed against workers using SCUBA from the surface, where times at the work site would be comparatively short, accompanied by periods of decompression before surfacing.

Thus began a series of experiments called SHAD (Shallow Habitat Air Diving) with Navy diver "volunteers." Two divers would live in a 9-foot across, 15-foot-long chamber for a month, undergoing a battery of physical, blood, and neuropsychological studies before entering the chamber. There was then further testing at the 50 (SHAD I) or 60-foot depth (SHAD II), when making deeper excursions (simulating work at depth), and after the final decompression. Air was supplied from a volume tank near the chamber. Emphasis was placed on the potential for the elevated partial pressure of oxygen to damage lung tissue, mandating extensive pulmonary function testing in the chamber.

This chamber had an outer lock which could be independently pressurized. On a near daily basis, I would enter the outer lock, be pressurized to the habitat depth, and enter the inner lock when the pressures between the two chambers were equalized, and a separating door could be opened. I performed physical exams, drew blood samples, and assessed general well-being, including psychological. Not unexpectedly, the divers became more cranky as the weeks wore on. They were, indeed, being put through their physical and mental paces. However, these experiments supported the premise that shallow habitat air diving with deeper excursions could be made safe and feasible.[23] As we planned for and conducted these experiments, my thoughts would occasionally wander back to the long hours of decompressing mice in that small room at Baylor where all of this started. The same considerations (compression and decompression profiles, the physiologic effects of the gases at elevated pressures, habitability) applied for both species.

The SHAD protocol was stressful for the divers, not least because of the confinement. In a different context, prolonged confinements are the normal routine for submariners. On the large nuclear- powered boats called "boomers," personnel are confined underwater for months at a time without surfacing. The intrigue of their missions is fascinating to read,[24] but their reality is an environment few could tolerate. All undergo thorough psychological vetting for this volunteer service. Physicians on the base were required to staff the hospital Emergency Room at nights and on weekends. On one of my shifts an enlisted man reported to the ER. He was visibly distraught. He told me his boat was scheduled to leave in the morning and that he could not do it; he could not "take it anymore." I thought the situation serious. I called the Commanding Officer of his boat, told him about his enlisted man's plea, and that I advised he not go on this patrol. The officer was sympathetic but indicated there was no replacement at this late hour and that my patient would go. I relayed the message. He was urged to seek help when the boat docked months later. I silently wished him well.

How would I do in a submarine? During the first year at the base, I had the opportunity to go aboard a submarine, a so-called fast attack boat. Officers on these boats would periodically invite the wives of their shipmates aboard this vessel as it went a short distance out to sea and submerged. When on these short outings a physician was required. I don't remember if I volunteered or was volunteered. All the while we were listening to one of officers explain shipboard living and the technologic devices that propel the sub and allow a habitable environment. Engagement with the surroundings and the explanations quickly overrode negative feelings. I suspect I could have adjusted to a long patrol on a submarine, though not at all comfortably.

A requirement for all Navy divers was an assessment of the individual's reaction to being in a dry chamber while compressed air was introduced to the equivalent of the pressure at 280 feet of sea water. The response under scrutiny was any adverse reaction to nitrogen narcosis due to the greatly elevated partial pressure of this gas. At this depth a "normal" response is one of subdued euphoria, even while unable to remember many personal details. The experience is truly mind altering. A physician was required on all these dives, often me. We were packed in a small chamber cheek to jowl, the latch closed, followed by the hissing of air entering the chamber. I was, of course, concerned the first time I squeezed into this small chamber. What if it was the physician who "flunked?" As the pressure increased the divers must be able to equalize the pressures in the middle ear, second nature to these men. The reaction to a brief stay at this depth must be unremarkable. The other divers and I negotiated these trials without incident. I am compelled to confess that air compressed to 280 feet is rather pleasant.

Just as divers had to prevail on this chamber dive, submariners had to "pass" a simulated escape from a submarine. I was often assigned to oversee these exercises in the 100-foot-tall submarine escape tower. If a submarine was to sink in relatively shallow water, personnel wearing a buoyant vest could enter a small compartment and "lock-out" at the pressure of the surrounding sea water. The vest, filled with air, would propel the person to the surface. During this ascent, air in the lungs must be continuously exhaled to avoid the risk that the air sacs would burst—as the pressure lessens during ascent the air in the lungs, initially compressed to the equivalent of 100 feet of sea water, would expand—with the high probability the bubbles escaping the lung would become lodged in the brain (an air embolism), causing a stroke. Fortunately, this is a rare occurrence and did not happen on my watch. A recompression chamber and an array of medications were on site to treat this malady. Air embolism can also result from any type of diving, from SCUBA to diving with mixed gases.

When the British submarine HMS *Thetis* sank while on sea trials in 1939, there were 103 men aboard. Only four were able to escape via the lock-out chamber. There were multiple failures, including a deterioration of air quality with a build-up of carbon dioxide. The government called upon J. B. S. Haldane to investigate. Haldane is one of the most intriguing and brilliant figures in the field of genetics.[25] Most of his work preceded the explosive knowledge in molecular details in recent decades. Beyond genetics, his interests, including politics, ranged broadly. He was an avowed communist, constantly under scrutiny by British intelligence services. As a scientist he had experimented on the physiological effects of gas composition on respiration; oxygen, carbon dioxide, helium, and nitrogen in various concentrations and under varying conditions of increased pressure and cold. Much of this experimentation was either self-administered or delivered into chambers at his direction. It often led to loss of consciousness, convulsions, and vomiting. It is this type of selfless (or foolhardy) experimentation Haldane and a few colleagues endured which catalyzed stringent efforts to maintain a safe environment for submariners.

The SHAD experiments continued, either in progress or planning the next, throughout my time in the lab. At a meeting during one of the SHAD trials, the Commanding Officer of the laboratory mentioned he had received a letter from a Dr. George Bass seeking a physician with diving experience, but more importantly a physician trained in Hyperbaric Medicine. I had developed the requisite knowledge base in this field during our experiments and at the diving school in D.C. This training would include the qualifications to treat cases of decompression sickness or air embolism in a chamber should the need arise. George, the acknowledged "father of underwater archeology," had been conducting underwater excavations of ancient shipwrecks in the Mediterranean Sea off the coast of Turkey. His work began in 1960, excavating a Bronze Age merchant vessel (dated to about 1200 BC) at Cape Gelidonya. This was the first underwater excavation completed in its entirety and to the same exacting standards employed by academics when excavating archeological sites on land.

When I was shown the letter, the contents stirred a powerful urge to be selected. It seemed a little quixotic and unlikely I could go. I knew George had sent this letter to all naval facilities employing physicians involved with diving activities. Also, I would first have to convince my Commanding Officer to allow me to go to Turkey for a period exceeding the allotted two weeks of vacation. If I succeeded in this endeavor, I would then have to lobby George. The shipwreck that was targeted for excavation in the summer of 1974 was at about one hundred feet. The usual procedure at that depth would be a morning work period of about twenty minutes at the site using SCUBA gear, a decompression period of between ten to fifteen minutes near the surface, with a repeat of this routine in the afternoon. This work schedule was clearly not efficient. I reasoned with the Commanding Officer that a SHAD-type of operation could greatly increase the efficiency of these excavations, and that I might be able to explore this with George as a "proof of principle." This reasoning carried the day.

I then attempted to contact George who was, at that time, living in Nicosia, Cyprus with his wife, Ann, and their two boys. I simultaneously ordered the National Geographic articles he had written about his work related to underwater archeology. After several tries, I was able to talk with him by phone and expressed my interest and background. He responded positively by mail about a week later. At the appointed time I went to Bodrum on the southwest coast of Turkey where George and his team (students, other professors, workers) stayed when not at an excavation site. In 1974 Bodrum was a small, sleepy village with a deep history, including the fifteenth-century construction of a castle at the entrance to the harbor. This Crusader castle, built by the Knights of St. John, was converted to the Bodrum Museum of Underwater Archeology in 1964 and now houses all the artifacts George and his team have recovered from these underwater excavations.

The goal of the 1974 campaign was a fourth-century AD Roman wreck which had struck a shallow reef off a small island called Yassi Ada. As further survey information became available, it was apparent that as many as 12 ships had struck this reef over millennia and sank. In addition to the Roman wreck, George and his team have excavated a seventh-century AD Byzantine wreck and a sixteenth-century AD Ottoman wreck at this site.

When I arrived, the relevant governmental agency had not yet issued a permit to do the work. George, who speaks fluent Turkish and was adept at negotiating the bureaucratic hurdles in Turkey, felt a trip to the capital, Ankara, was required to discuss the delay with officials. I rode with him. We were able to establish a quick rapport. He told me about his family, and I shared a little about mine. We also discussed the SHAD work at the submarine base. George was a voracious reader, a skilled orator, and an accomplished author. He was enterprising and inventive. Many of the techniques that allow recovery of artifacts sequestered on the ocean floor for centuries were pioneered by George and his colleagues. For a time in the 1960s he even had a submersible submarine manufactured by General Dynamics Electric Boat to assist his efforts. He had already considered shallow habitat air diving as a means to enhance efficiency. Had I known him better, this revelation would not have been at all surprising. This trip was the beginning of a warm relationship with George and Ann.

The project began in earnest when the necessary paperwork arrived. Diving operations commenced from a barge carrying a recompression chamber to treat cases of decompression sickness. Tanks of compressed air were connected to the chamber, and oxygen was available as needed. We (yes, George allowed physicians to participate as working divers) had been working for about two weeks when a Turkish naval vessel appeared. An officer told us a war had started on Cyprus between the Turks living in the north and the Greeks occupying the south of this country. He ordered us to return to the mainland. We retreated to a small village on the coast. The fear of a wider war engulfing the mainland was quite real. After two weeks the situation calmed, and I returned to the states. My continued friendship with the Basses and association with the Institute of Nautical Archeology, founded by George and several of his colleagues, have been sources of real companionship and intellectual stimulation.

Shortly after I returned from Turkey, I was talking to one of the administrators in the laboratory who belonged to the Navy Flying Club. As it happened, he headed the membership committee. When I expressed more than casual interest, he arranged a meeting with one of the flight instructors. I had previously read about a group in Africa, the East African Flying Physician Service, and fantasized myself in the cockpit of one of their aircraft, flying to remote areas to delivery urgent care to isolated villages. I began to take lessons in a small aircraft, a Cessna 150. As with diving or almost any endeavor which took me out of a cocooned, well-structured routine, I approached flying, despite its allure, with a measure of trepidation. I negotiated the lessons reasonably well, soloing relatively early in the process, thereby gaining confidence. However, I could not overcome my uncertainty, and did not complete the certification, reasoning that I would do so later, particularly if it could be combined with the provision of medical care. Later in life I did return to flying lessons, though not in preparation for medical work in Africa.

Over many years, as I have read and thought about the scientific subject matter I hope can serve as a reciprocal complement to this personal narrative, I have reflected that endeavors like diving and flying can foster thinking on a more expansive scale. Participation in these activities had this effect on me. Beginning with the hyperbaric work at Baylor, I immersed myself in the literature, trying to obtain a "sense" for the sheer physical reality of the increasing pressure down the water column of the oceans, the crushing pressures at the deepest trenches, yet even at great depths ecosystems populated with an array of organisms are encountered, as are ocean floor vents which hold within them the possibility for the origin of life. Sonar has mapped the bottom contours, and remotely operated vehicles have acted as our "eyes" to view these unexplored regions. Submersibles have ferried aquanauts to the extremities of the ocean floor. Indeed, a great variety of conveyances, some of them now quirky curiosities, have transported brave men and women into that dark realm, propelled by ingenuity and inquisitiveness. On a more mundane level, diving also brings attention to the gas laws and the physiologic consequences of elevated or lowered partial pressure of these gases. These features, and so many more, are touchstones of a deeper view.

The transition at water's surface enormously expands this view, a transition to a medium (air) which has sustained life on land through an intricate balance of adaptations over eons. The decreasing pressure up through the layers of the atmosphere and the vast beyond, the spacecraft, the probes, the instruments collecting information, most remarkably the telescopes, the possibility of life elsewhere in the cosmos and, again, the brave men and women who dare to go forth, all of these and more excite the imagination and a desire to know more. As a smart book has amply and poetically documented, when mind co-mingles with the cosmos a more vivid reality emerges.[26]

As has been mentioned, the pursuit of external goals like flying and diving has been consuming. These goals and those associated with an academic career have also been anxiety generating. This clash has been a constant struggle. The drive to reach a goal has usually held sway, not so much by swamping anxiety as by forcing an uneasy accommodation of two powerful forces. How this accommodation has been achieved is beyond my poor powers to understand or articulate. However, I have appreciated that intellectual gain has been a feature of this tradeoff.

Against this backdrop of work and rumination, I began to ponder a career path. I knew I could continue in the Navy, but early in the process I eliminated this as a possibility. I would pursue more medical training. My last rotation in medical school, as mentioned, had been Ob/Gyn. Without exposure to this specialty, it was not in the running when I had to choose an internship. As I reflected, I found much to like about Ob/Gyn as a student and began to seriously consider it as a life's work, ultimately getting to an affirmative answer. It was then a matter of applying to programs. My preference, if it could be arranged, was to enter at the second year of the four-year training program, having already completed an internship. I was fortunate there was an opening to start the second year at the University of New Mexico School of Medicine program in Albuquerque. I was accepted and would start in July 1975.

At the end of my Navy service, I had a few months before residency would begin. As stated above, I wanted to investigate the possibility of one day going to East Africa and working with the East Africa Flying Doctor Services, founded in 1957 by a British surgeon, Dr. Michael Wood. It happened he would be speaking at a symposium in Nairobi, Kenya organized by

International Seminars. The trip was scheduled. Following a stop in Rabat, Morocco for tours and medical lectures, I flew to Nairobi. After settling into a hotel, I went back to Nairobi's Wilson Airport where I knew the flying physician's organization had a new hangar for their aircraft. I walked over to the facility and saw a small woman I recognized from photographs to be Dr. Anne Spoerry. She was born in France in 1918 and had been a medical practitioner in East Africa since 1951. At the time she joined the flying group in 1965, she was one of five physicians. Two, including her, flew their own planes. I introduced myself and told her my interest. She projected purpose and strength. She suggested I talk to Dr. Wood, which I had planned to do after the upcoming seminar.

Indeed, following Dr. Wood's presentation I engaged him. He was attentive and forthright. He inquired how long I would be willing to commit. I had envisioned one or two years following residency. He stood erect and began, in a non-judgmental way, to explain that their need was for a long-term commitment, ideally a career. He was not in any way lecturing or chastising. He expressed gratitude for my interest, which seemed to end our conversation. At that moment I was humbled; I acutely realized this plan of mine was born of overweening ambition. A year or two to have an "experience" would not do much to improve the health of the region. I have tried since that time, not always successfully, to be aware that hubris, often a cover for other inadequacies, can be a malign motivating force. However, this brush with the provision of care to needy citizens of the world helped fuel a continued interest in international health. (Following retirement, I experienced a hands-on sense for the vast scope of this undertaking when I joined a local medical group going to Haiti.)

Though the mental demons were not as punishing during this stint in the Navy as they had been in the past, the depression and anxiety I had experienced nonetheless continued. Dysphoric feelings sparked by any number of triggers, inner and outer, still held the ground for a significant fraction of the day and often the night. Panicky feelings were sometimes a part of this mix. Despite my experience at Baylor, I was ready to again seek help, to give talk therapy another chance. Though I was loathe to discuss these issues with others, an officer on the base I trusted, who had obtained a medical degree at Yale, suggested a psychotherapist with ties to this institution. His home/office was in the Connecticut countryside, an easy drive from

Groton. I went there once a week for about a year. My Navy salary, though far from a princely sum, was just adequate to live on and afford the therapy.

Though I did not make great strides in psychotherapy, the sessions did spark insights I could use in the future. At that time, however, I was still concentrating on future goals in a self-absorbed manner, relegating a relationship which had developed to a secondary status. My behavior was akin to that I have decried in my father. I was focused on the upcoming Ob/Gyn residency, knowing it would be another intense period of full-time attention to work and learning. It would also bring another relationship, one which would call upon all the psychological guard rails I had struggled to construct.

§§§

WHILE STILL in the Navy prior to beginning residency training, George Bass called to ask if I would participate in another underwater excavation in the Aegean Sea. I explained I was moving to Albuquerque, but that Tim was an accomplished SCUBA diver, could competently treat diving related illnesses and accidents, and would surely bring himself up to speed on any deficiencies. Tim was able to go for two consecutive summers, and even treated a Turkish sponge diver with a severe case of decompression sickness brought to the excavation site where his fellow divers knew there would be a recompression chamber.

Entering at the second year of a four-year residency, I had to scramble to fill the knowledge and experience gap. The University of New Mexico School of Medicine had recruited Dr. Robert Messer to be Chair of the department, a man with a deep commitment to the educational development of his charges. He, in turn, had recruited key faculty members, including those with training in the subdisciplines of reproductive endocrinology and gynecologic oncology. The residency was, of course, arduous and emotionally demanding. However, the cultural diversity of the patient population helped to offset the grind. A large fraction of patients was Hispanic and Native American from the numerous tribes and pueblos (mostly Pueblo, but also Zuni, Navajo, and others). Many came from groups whose healing traditions made our jobs more challenging, but immensely interesting.

The program provided a wealth of patient experience to hone judgment and skills; the judgment to discern the optimal method to safely deliver a baby in individual cases, and the skills to do so. Gynecological surgery also demanded judgment and a set of skills learned from many hours in the operating room with accomplished mentors. The oncology service was particularly demanding, but greatly expanded a resident's comfort with surgical technique. Some of the ovarian cancer surgeries, with residents usually serving as assistants, were multi-hour marathons. As residency progressed, I slowly gained a hard-won confidence, born of lessons imparted by supervisory staff and, most critically, fellow residents more senior than me.

One particularly difficult duty required of the four of us at the second-year level was the management of rape cases brought to the Emergency Room; taking the detailed history, performing the examination, and, lastly, handing the labeled evidence from the genital examination to police outside the room to assure there was no break in the chain of evidence. If necessary, we were also called to testify in court. These cases compel sensitivity and compassion. A three-year-old girl was brought in by her mother. She sat on the edge of the examining table, staring blankly ahead, with an occasional soft whimper. After the preliminaries, a quick glance revealed a large vaginal tear. She was taken to the operating room where the tear was repaired, and the crime evidence collected. Months later, when I entered the room of an 83-year-old woman who had been brutally raped, I noted the same blank stare, trying to bring her attention to what had happened to her, expressing uncomprehending disbelief in a barely audible voice.

At some point during my second year in Albuquerque, dad reappeared. He was drawn to the diverse cultures, art, and beauty of Santa Fe, a charming city in northern New Mexico. His plans were unformed, but he had rented a dwelling, suggesting to me he was going to be there for a time. He found employment as a waiter in a counter-cultural vegetarian restaurant, one harkening back to the 1960s. I suspect his age, largely traditional thinking, and ordinary clothing did not easily mesh with the owners and other employees, but he seemed enthused to be in this setting.

After he settled in, he called, indicating he would be coming to Albuquerque and could we go out to eat? During the conversation over dinner, he announced he was a recent convert to Catholicism. His tone of seriousness suggested he had fully embraced this religion and the entirety of its teachings. It soon became evident he had a mission for this trip, one related to his conversion. Over my lifetime he had made only a few suggestions to me, such as his perceived benefit of my joining a college fraternity. The subject he now broached was of a much more serious nature. He seemed determined to extract a promise that I not perform abortions. These procedures were legal at that time and training was provided in residency, though a resident was obviously not required to perform these procedures. I was wholly unprepared for this sudden swerve in our conversation. I sensed he anticipated a response. A leaden quiet hung over the table. I remained frozen. After an interminable passage of time, a less freighted topic thankfully ensued. The subject of abortion was never again discussed.

Dad continued working in the restaurant and joined a local church and its choir, thus allowing him to indulge one of his passions, singing. He also took seriously the Christian duty to provide for others. I drove to Santa Fe one weekend to find him in the kitchen preparing meals-on-wheels to distribute to shut-ins. I helped him carry the food to the car and drove with him. He seemed on edge, apparently concerned that his offerings would be well received. As we pulled out of the driveway, he drove over a deep rut beside the driveway he had obviously forgotten was there. Some of the containers of hot food on the floor mats tumbled over, spilling their contents. He was very dismayed. In that moment I felt compassion for him.

When I next heard from him, he had decided to buy a small mobile home and had relocated to a trailer park in Tesuque, just outside of Santa Fe. Within just a few months of this move he informed me of yet another major transition: he was going to become a monk. He had petitioned and been accepted into the Benedictine Monastery (Our Lady of Guadalupe Abbey) in Pecos, 25 miles east of Santa Fe. Though curious, I never explored with him the mental machinations that led to this decision and the requirements he had to satisfy to begin his quest into this Catholic religious order with deep roots in Bavaria and Switzerland.[27]

I drove to the monastery one weekend day in late summer/early fall. A few miles outside Pecos I turned into the entrance and noted the scent of pine tree forests and the achingly blue sky. Down from the outbuildings flanking the central Abbey were gardens, and beyond was the smooth flowing Pecos River, serene beneath the far bluff. A duck pond sporting several species of birds was nearby. Before seeing him, I walked the path by the river for a short distance. I felt comforted by the setting. This initially prepared me to look charitably upon his decision.

When I was shown to his single room in the dormitory with radiant light streaming through the window, he was resting on his bed which occupied, I estimate, about one quarter of the room's space. A lamp and radio were on a bedside stand, a small rug, basin, bureau, and a potted plant the remaining articles. As he showed me around, he spoke glowingly of this monastic life he had chosen. He introduced me to others in his newfound circle, all warm and positive people. As the day passed, I gradually developed the conviction that dad was in his element and that he needed this ordered structure (though he would have chafed at this suggestion). I was gratified that his attempts to counter his sometimes chaotic, sometimes desperately unhappy life had brought him to this sanctuary with the promise of inner and outer tranquility.

That night I stayed for their singing. Shortly, a disquieting ceremony occurred. A teenage girl was brought by friends and family to the room filled with singing congregants. A group of them pressed toward her, arms upraised, singing and chanting, my father among them. The girl, terrified, then screaming, bolted from the room and ran into the forest. I learned she was schizophrenic; her condition had not responded to more conventional therapies.

Thus, I came to know about the tradition of healing in some monasteries. I was disappointed that dad, with the training he had received, including a year in psychiatry residency before quitting, was a participant in an exercise that, at least on this evening, had likely exacerbated this girl's illness. When he indicated he was going to be a monk he was obviously a committed novitiate, as demonstrated by the events of this evening. I got in my car and drove the several hours back to Albuquerque, reflecting on this eventful day.

I continued to believe dad had found a good emotional fit for what I assumed would be the remainder of his life. But no. He had entered the monastery in the summer. I drove up for the last time that winter. We motored to a Pecos establishment, ordered a hot beverage, and stood beside a wood burning stove. This is when he let it be known he had "met" Bill and produced a letter from him with the closing Your Loving Bill. How they met I don't know. This was years before the internet. Dad had decided they would move to Rye, the small village where he had such fond childhood memories. The chance to recapture some of this old magic with a new mate proved irresistible. They would begin a life together in an older, small home on a sparse plot of land with a horse corral.

Soon after dad had thrown in his lot with monastic life, I returned to the Labor and Delivery suite in the early morning hours after a consultation in the Emergency Room. I noted the white board with all the laboring patients, including such particulars as how dilated the patient's cervix was, along with other pertinent information. A female medical student was at the desk writing a note in one of the charts. At the end of her Ob/Gyn rotation she began a conversation and asked if I would like to go to a movie with her. Nancy was personable and attractive. We went to a movie, the start of a relationship, and after several dates I was smitten. She was the eldest of 10 children in a close family. I was comforted by the warm, supportive environment when we visited her family in northern New Mexico.

Perhaps two months into the relationship she said she had experienced some discomfort in her lower abdomen and had felt a mass in this region. I felt the same firm mass rising above the pelvic bone. This obviously required medical attention. She was seen by Dr. Robert Hilgers, the department's gynecologic oncologist. A work-up suggested this mass was arising from the left ovary. At surgery Dr. Hilgers removed the tumor along with the left ovary. The immediate concern was cancer. A preliminary pathology report while the operation continued was inconclusive, so the uterus and other ovary were not removed and a more extensive intra-abdominal surgery was not performed, as would occur when the operating room diagnosis is ovarian cancer.

As sometimes happens in medicine, a definitive diagnosis can sometimes be difficult to declare, with disagreement among experts, particularly if a disease (or tumor) is rare. Dr. Hilgers, in addition to extra years of training to become a certified gynecologic oncologist, had also completed an extra year of training in pathology related to gynecologic tumors. He concluded, after his evaluation of the slides under the microscope, that the tumor was malignant. He sent slides to experts he had trained with. The consensus was that this tumor was a malignant fibrosarcoma.

"Sarcoma" is a dread term in medicine. These are often very aggressive and can arise from many sites in the body. Nancy would be administered chemotherapy. The hair loss, nausea and vomiting, the external effects, would be accompanied by what patients tell us about the internal, more hidden effects; the fatigue, worsening of depression and anxiety which inevitably accompany the diagnosis of cancer, and the mental fog and cognitive impairment. Nancy continued her rotations on the ward, but grew increasingly depressed, not uncommon for someone in her situation. She had been a "take charge" individual, providing much of the care for her younger siblings. Becoming so dependent upon others was only one of the multiple challenges she faced.

I began to administer chemotherapy at her home by IV infusion to avoid hospitalizations for these treatments, as was done at that time. As these courses of chemotherapy progressed her depression deepened. Her verbalizations became more threatening. I steeled myself against the possibility she may harm herself or worse and responded with all the verbal suasion, understanding, and physical closeness I was capable of. When other circumstances supervened I could tell, despite efforts to counter it, that the emotional ground had shifted and my affection was in subtle retreat. With her heightened senses on guard for any form of threat, she had to have known this also. Fortunately, she improved as she finished her courses of chemotherapy, and, against the odds, she completed medical school with her original classmates. She had overcome with a grim determination.

In the meantime, residency training inexorably marched on. I had earlier indicated that the chairman, Dr. Messer, had recruited a talented faculty representing all the extant subspecialties. This group of subspecialists included Marshall Levine. At that time, he was only the fourth obstetrician in the U.S. to receive two years of Fellowship training in Medical Genetics beyond residency. Most of the early trainees in this field were pediatricians. This made sense; 3 percent of all newborns have a birth defect or defects (ranging from minor to severe), and genetic counseling is indicated in these cases. The field was broadened when prenatal testing of a fetus became feasible with the advent of ultrasound imaging and amniocentesis, the insertion of a needle into the fluid surrounding the fetus to collect fetal cells. These can be used to analyze the chromosomes in these cells under a microscope.

As I listened to Dr. Levine counsel a patient or couple and observed him perform amniocenteses, I became quite taken with Medical Genetics as applied to obstetrics. Most patients were referred for a maternal age indication, given the association between increasing age of the mother and delivery of a child with 47 chromosomes (Down syndrome and several others) rather than the normal 46. There were many other reasons a patient may be referred to Dr. Levine, such as previous delivery of a child with a birth defect.

From its inception, training in Medical Genetics emphasized a cardinal principle: the counseling must be non-directive. The facts and options must be clearly conveyed so decisions can be based on solid information. This decision-making process cannot be contravened by the substituted judgment of the physician. The counselor must take as long as necessary, scheduling additional sessions if required for understanding. Though ultrasound at that time produced fetal images vastly inferior to those available now, I was present for several sessions when Dr. Levine was counseling a couple following the discovery of a severe fetal malformation by ultrasound. These intense sessions required a large knowledge base and the deepest sensitivity. Genetic counseling is the bedrock.

Dr. Levine transmitted his enthusiasm for genetics. Writ large, the increasingly sophisticated understanding of genetics provided a more nuanced picture of evolution. In medicine, genetics was opening a window on disease processes at the molecular level. The expectation that genetics applied to obstetrics would become a burgeoning field with development of newer techniques and laboratory advances, coupled with improved methods to image fetuses had captivated me. These advancements could lead to more accurate diagnosis of a range of fetal conditions, as well as the prospect of fetal treatments for some. However, at that time no one could envision the rapidity of these advances. With about eight months remaining in residency, I told Dr. Levine I wished to pursue a Medical Genetics Fellowship. He seemed pleased; he had obviously had an impact. Had his example not been before me, it is unlikely I would have engaged this further training.

I applied to two programs, one in Los Angeles at the Cedars-Sinai Medical Center where Dr. Levine had trained, and one in San Francisco with Mitchell Golbus, an obstetrical geneticist who was building a strong prenatal testing program. I was accepted to both, and initially elected to go to LA. This program employed one of the handful of obstetricians, Dr. Lawrence Karp, specifically trained in Medical Genetics, though he did not overlap Dr. Levine's time there. Within weeks after accepting the Cedars-Sinai offer I learned Dr. Karp was going to join the faculty at the University of Washington School of Medicine in Seattle. The certainty that the presence of Dr. Karp on the faculty would enhance my experience led me to call him to inquire about the possibility of training in Seattle. He suggested I call Dr. Judith Hall, the Fellowship director. She was welcoming on the telephone. She indicated that the training positions had been filled, but also allowed that she and many of her pediatric colleagues were eager to have more obstetricians in the field. She would talk to Dr. Arno Motulsky, head of the Genetics Division, and he consented. He could free up funds from his National Institutes of Health Training Grant to support an additional trainee.

I would spend the next two years, 1978–1980, in Seattle. The lure of the northwest and reputation of the medical school and this specific training program seemed to bode well. It had been the school where Tim, several years previously, had received his MD and PhD in neurophysiology, productive of two solid publications in a respected journal.[28, 29] Nancy's follow-up tests showed no evidence of a recurrence of her ovarian cancer. Her mood had stabilized, her blond hair had grown out, and she began to display the determination and seeming confidence she had before her illness. She desired a continuing relationship, but also wanted to become an Emergency Room physician, requiring a two-year residency to become fully certified in this specialty. She was selected by the University of Colorado program in Denver.

⁛

THIS PERIOD of life, a Medical Genetics Fellowship, was dominated by the accumulating knowledge base in genetics and by close association, via mentoring, with many leaders in the field. Two of the towering figures in medical genetics, Dr. Victor McKusick and Dr. Arno Motulsky, had anticipated that the explanatory power of genetics would place this field at the forefront of medical knowledge and research. In 1957, these luminaries founded bicoastal departments of Medical Genetics within their respective departments of medicine, Dr. McKusick at Johns Hopkins University and Dr. Motulsky at the University of Washington.

Dr. Motulsky's story is a harrowing one. After a happy childhood in East Prussia, then a part of Germany, his family saw the looming Nazi threat as WWII approached. He was a passenger on the German liner *St. Louis* with 1,100 Jewish refugees bound for coveted freedom. As the world watched, the ship was turned back at Cuba and refused entry into America when the ship passed the Miami area. After the vessel's return to Europe Dr. Motulsky survived several threats to his life, ultimately made it to America, and became a physician. He developed expertise in hematology (blood disorders) at several centers. He began his academic career in Seattle in 1953, the year James Watson and Francis Crick discovered the double-helical structure of DNA. When he taught, he would "bootleg"—as he liked to assert—genetic aspects of hematology into his student lectures. This emphasis on the hereditary nature of many disorders led his department chairman to suggest he start a Genetics Division.

Dr. Motulsky's storied career led him in multiple directions. Based on many lines of evidence, including his pioneering studies, he realized drugs could be differentially metabolized based on an individual's genetic make-up. He was the first to propose the term "pharmacogenetics," a field which has been a harbinger of the anticipated era of personalized medicine.[30] He was keenly interested in Jewish genetics, the study of genetic diseases found in greater numbers in Jewish populations and the reason(s) this may be so. He fostered collegiality. It is not a surprise that a major text in human genetics was co-authored by Dr. Motulsky and a German geneticist, Friedrich Vogel. Many of his trainees have had distinguished careers, including Nobel Prize winner Joe Goldstein. Toward the end of his life Dr. Motulsky related his early history and his career to another notable geneticist, Dr. Mary-Claire King.[30]

Judith Hall, who facilitated my acceptance into the fellowship, was a medical student at the University of Washington when she became captivated by this "new" field, so much so that she chose an extra year of medical school to pursue a master's degree in genetics under the tutelage of Dr. Motulsky. Following medical school, she completed training in pediatrics at John Hopkins where she was a co-intern with Dr. James Hanson, who became head of Medical Genetics at the University of Iowa Medical School. She continued her interest in genetics under Dr. McKusick when she was accepted into the two-year Genetics Fellowship he directed. Her subsequent career as a clinician, educator, clinical researcher, department chair, and leader in many other capacities during a time genetics assumed its pivotal role in medicine and the biosciences, is deserving of enduring respect.[31] I remember her for her immense energy, productivity, and warmth.

Dr. Hall was an astute and sensitive clinical observer. If a child had a birth defect or defects, a myriad of questions were pondered: what was the mechanism(s) by which these defects arose; when, in development, did they begin to manifest; what is the usual course these problems take; how do they impact the child socially and emotionally; and so many other issues she would pursue in the course of evaluation of the child and counseling the parents. She took as her areas of expertise the range of developmental disabilities but is perhaps most closely identified with her interest in dwarfing conditions, those producing short stature. She published widely in this field and was a revered, and readily accessible, figure within the alliance group called Little People of America.

Her interest in understanding the trajectory of these disorders—how they change over time and with what consequences for the individual—led she and Dr. Virginia Sybert to start a clinic, in which I participated, to address these questions for a condition called Turner syndrome, most commonly caused by the absence of one of the X chromosomes in females. The X and Y are the sex-determining chromosomes, females having two Xs and males a single X and Y. Girls and women with Turner syndrome have short stature, have other more minor physical features, and are infertile because their ovaries do not develop. Mental retardation is not a feature of Turner syndrome. However, to truly understand the health consequences of Turner syndrome over a lifetime, longitudinal studies are required.[32] This applies to many conditions seen in a genetics clinic, as Dr. Hall realized.

In addition to Drs. Motulsky and Hall, there were many bright and dedicated faculty to which those of us in the Fellowship had access. The overriding goals for this training were to become knowledgeable about the multiple mechanisms by which a person's genetic endowment and environment can cause or contribute to a vast number of conditions, to become proficient at identifying these disease states, and to accurately counsel patients and their families about all aspects of the condition and the implications, reproductive and otherwise, for family members. Prior to seeing these patients, an accurate family pedigree, including relevant medical histories, was imperative.

Fellows in training came from varied backgrounds and would pursue varied career paths. Therefore, our clinical experience was tailored to match our career plans. Because I came from obstetrical training, I attended prenatal diagnosis clinics at the main teaching hospital and Swedish hospital, affiliated with the medical school. This clinic was staffed by Dr. Lawrence Karp, previously mentioned as having recently moved from a faculty position at a medical school in Los Angeles. The expertise to be gained in these clinics was performing amniocentesis procedures, to become proficient at interpreting ultrasound images of fetuses, and counseling patients about the reason for their referral, and, if a fetal abnormality was detected, the implications of this finding(s). Many of these referrals were for maternal age greater than 35 with an increased chance to conceive a child with a chromosome abnormality such as an extra chromosome number 21, which results in Down syndrome, and other chromosome imbalances. Other reasons for referral may include concern about a fetal abnormality detected on ultrasound and delivery of a child with a condition which may recur in a subsequent pregnancy, and which would be amenable to detection by amniocentesis and/or ultrasound.

Though I had not met Larry Karp prior to my arrival in Seattle, he had considerable influence on my thinking and approach to the field of medical genetics. He was unassuming and somewhat shy, with an artistic temperament. He stuttered, most noticeably and painfully when counseling patients. His eyes would close, his contorted face straining at the effort he was making to bring a word or thought forward. Patients seemed initially discomfited, but when they realized his persistent effort betrayed an earnest attempt to provide them comprehensive information, they seemed to merge their vulnerabilities at that moment with his. They were in it together.

Dr. Karp has written numerous books, including an early one on genetic engineering.[33] A prior book reflected his experiences as an intern at Bellevue Hospital in New York City,[34] the hospital of last resort for the sick and unfortunate. Bellevue has a history I could understand.[35] Tales of the sort offered by historical accounts of Bellevue are reminiscent of the experiences I had as a medical student and intern in the Emergency Room of the Ben Taub city-county hospital in Houston. Dr. Karp's novel well describes the setting, the excessive work, and the patients in memorable, tragicomic vignettes. The schedule, typical for the time, was brutal; on (in the hospital) every other night, in addition to daytime duties. As he described in the book, after many exhausting months of this routine, he had a temporary "break" with reality and was sent to his apartment to catch up on sleep and reconnect with the world.

Dr. Karp was articulate and thoughtful. His ruminations on the ethical challenges presented by genetics, and perhaps most acutely by reproductive issues, coupled with his writing skills, attracted the attention of another very accomplished geneticist of the era, Dr. John Opitz, the editor of the *American Journal of Human Genetics*. By mutual agreement, Dr. Karp would pen short columns in this journal under the rubric *Genetic Drift* to highlight areas of genetics with profound ethical implications: abortion, eugenics, sterilization of the retarded, and so many others. Dr. Opitz did not constrain the message; these pieces were not bound by the usual, staid academic formulae. They were literary expressions, liberal in outlook, and sometimes quite edgy.[36]

In another *Genetic Drift* offering, Dr. Karp paid tribute to a larger-than-life figure in genetics who had also found an academic home in Seattle, Dr. David Smith, written a day after his death.[37] Dr. Smith founded the field of dysmorphology, a term he coined in 1966, referring to the study of human congenital defects or those which occur prior to birth. He was an affable, large man with a generous spirit and a ready, wide smile. In addition to our other clinics, Fellows were assigned a short rotation through Dr. Smith's clinic. I well remember the late afternoon he was called to counsel a couple who had just delivered a baby with Down syndrome at a hospital on the periphery of Seattle. I joined him as we drove to the site. In a grandfatherly manner, he established an easy and immediate rapport with the young, anxious couple before turning his full attention on the baby. After a long give-and-take counseling session, during which his natural, sunny outlook almost willed a bonding between the parents and their baby with his realistic, but generally positive, words about the potential for Down syndrome children, the anxious demeanors the couple initially displayed were replaced by a more hopeful outlook.

David Smith was head of a training program in the field he founded. Many of his Fellows became leaders at other institutions, including the previously mentioned Dr. James Hanson, who joined the faculty in Iowa City. Dr. Hanson, with Dr. Smith, made seminal observations in the field of teratology, the study of abnormal fetal development caused by medications and other exogenous or environmental agents which can harm a fetus, a field intimately linked with dysmorphology. They described, for example, the Fetal Hydantoin Syndrome caused by the anticonvulsant Dilantin.[38]

In addition to our clinical work, Fellows in training were expected to conduct research, either laboratory or clinical. The head of the department of Ob/Gyn, Dr. Morton Stenchever, had established a laboratory which performed studies on gametes, sperm and eggs or ova. Dr. Karp was also involved with this research. After a discussion with him and Dr. Stenchever, the expectation that I would work in this laboratory seemed certain, and so it was. When I reported to the lab, the technician described the principal project, a test of male fertility called the sperm penetration assay (SPA). Eggs retrieved from female hamsters were placed in a petri dish with appropriate media. The outer covering of the eggs, the zona pellucida, was chemically removed. This structure facilitates entry of human sperm into human eggs but proved a barrier to entry into hamster ova. After the appropriate period of interaction among the sperm and hamster ova, the percent of eggs which sperm had penetrated was tallied. In early studies, the SPA seemed to discriminate males of infertile couples in which a "male factor" was the issue.[39] Over time and with more experimentation, this test was shown to be insufficiently predictive to be useful in routine clinical practice.

We also had access to sperm which were completely immotile; these cells showed no movement owing to structural defects in the tails (the motive force) of these cells. Motility is required for human sperm to fertilize human ova. I placed these sperm with tail defects into a dish with the hamster ova without zona pellucidae, thinking sperm penetration could not possibly occur without movement. To our surprise, the eggs were able to incorporate these sperm into the cell interior in numbers comparable to tests with motile sperm.[40] At least in this system, the egg was more than a passive recipient.

My time was divided among general genetics clinics, laboratory work, and prenatal diagnostic clinics. Though this period of training was several years prior to the advent of fetal surgery, even now rarely performed, several advancements anticipated the development of fetal surgery. One advancement was a technique called fetoscopy wherein a thin tube, a fetoscope, was inserted through the uterus and into the amniotic fluid. The fetus could be directly visualized to verify defects suspected on ultrasound, and, through a side port, blood could be drawn and tissues biopsied to determine if the fetus did or did not have a serious genetic disease for which the fetus was at risk. This procedure was associated with a heightened risk of pregnancy loss over a procedure such as amniocentesis. However, it was a skill a person with my training would seriously consider acquiring at that time. This would require travel to a center specializing in the technique. I started with a physician at Yale. I called him, expressing my desire to learn fetoscopy from him. He answered in the affirmative and we settled on a date. I arrived on the east coast and found a motel in New Haven. At the appointed time the following day I went to his clinic and encountered his assistant, a non-physician who was apparently in charge of his daily routine. I told her why I was there and presented relevant correspondence. She gruffly said the physician was out of town, there were other visiting physicians, and bluntly ended the conversation by uttering "we can't possibly accommodate you." I resignedly drove back to the motel, reflecting on this disappointment, repeatedly telling myself to avoid the trap of becoming so self-important (and busy) that I could let an episode like this happen on my watch.

When time availed, I read books outside my field of training, often those related to the functioning of the brain. Years earlier I had slogged through Freud's *Interpretation of Dreams,* perhaps trying to understand the therapeutic task of analysis and why I had failed so miserably during my stint on the couch. The book was highly imaginative but produced no clarity. I was not expected back in Seattle for several days, so began reading a large tome which convincingly argued that Freud, with his initial background as a neurologist, fundamentally believed that psychiatric disorders were caused by altered brain biology.[41] In my far from fully formed musings on this subject, I sensed that this was the case. Freud was influenced by Darwin and other contemporary scholars, countering the notion that all his insights came from his daunting self-analysis. However, it was gratifying to learn that this maverick genius held a biological perspective. Somehow this helped salvage an otherwise fruitless trip.

Toward the end of the two-year Fellowship, it was time to apply for an academic job at a school of medicine. Before this process began in earnest, Dr. Stenchever approached me to offer a position in his department. I was pleased, knowing that faculty positions in this medical school were coveted. I also surmised he likely anticipated I would continue research in his laboratory, at least for a time, research from which he was quite removed. Another drawback was the weather in the northwest. No sunlight for days on end during the winter months clearly exacerbated the dogged depression.

After the interview process was completed, I received desirable offers from academic medical institutions whose Ob/Gyn department chairmen had realized that genetics could have a positive impact on their fields, as this discipline had demonstrated in other fields of medicine. Ultimately, I elected to join the faculty in Iowa City. Nancy had also interviewed for a faculty position in the ER Department and received a favorable response. The Ob/Gyn department had maintained a good national reputation, and the institution had a strong research base. Dr. James Hanson, head of the Division of Genetics within the Department of Pediatrics and a trainee of Dr. David Smith in Seattle, had a big influence on my decision. I was impressed with his public health perspective, partnering with state health agencies to legislatively mandate a single, centralized, not-for-profit laboratory to perform the genetic screening tests, those on newborns and those under consideration for pregnant women. When this latter aspect of genetic screening was realized, I would direct this statewide program. Other, more peripheral reasons influenced my decision. The chairman of the Department of Psychiatry, Dr. George Winokur, had been among the few leaders at that time advocating that the foundation of this field should be genetics and biology. This seemed an enlightened position that would improve the overall intellectual environment at the school. One of Dr. Winokur's faculty members, Dr. Nancy Andreasen, was also becoming well-known as an early advocate for studying psychiatric diseases from a biological perspective,[42] for her imaging studies of the brains of patients with disorders such as schizophrenia, and her interest in the link between mood disorders and creativity. Her PhD in English and past association with the Iowa Writers' Workshop honed her skills as a talented writer. She received the National Medal of Science from President Clinton in 2000.

The medical school in Iowa City has had a tradition of support for women in medicine, including leadership positions. The institution was founded in 1870, then called The University of Iowa Medical Department. Thirty-seven students were admitted to the first class, eight of whom were women, one of the first coeducational medical schools in the nation. I also made a mental note that Tennessee Williams had received a BA in Theater Arts at Iowa in 1938. A major life experience was acting in one of his plays in high school. Williams, I later learned, worked as a waiter in the doctor's dining area at University Hospitals. I was unwittingly attaching some significance to these connections, mere coincidences, as we are wont to do. It pleased me to note that shortly after I began employment at University

Hospitals in 1981, the formalized segregation of dining areas ceased. In many ways medicine has become more egalitarian.

It also did not hurt that there was much happening at the undergraduate school across the Iowa River from the medical school. Iowa had won 15 national wrestling titles under their legendary coach Dan Gable. My ardor for the sport has waned somewhat, but I still have admiration for these athletes and the sacrifices required to be competitive. The gymnastics team was always competitive. I was also aware that the renowned Iowa Writers' Workshop brought legions of notable authors to town to read from their work, though at that time I had no aspiration to write. Iowa City was subsequently designated a City of Literature by UNESCO, the first city in the U.S. to receive this designation, and only the third worldwide at that time. I was also made aware of the many significant contributions to space exploration by members of the physics department under their folksy chair who grew up just down the road from Iowa City, Dr. James Van Allen,[43] discoverer of the Van Allen radiation belts. Over the years, investigators from that department have placed instrumentation aboard many space craft which have had a major impact on the stunning discoveries made in space. The plasma wave instrument, developed in the physics department, was critical in determining that the Voyager I spacecraft, launched in 1977, had flown beyond the confines of our solar system after 36 years in flight![44, 45] Voyager II is now also in interstellar space. Remarkably, both are still transmitting data as I write this.

I went to Denver following Fellowship to join Nancy. Though there was a chance our relationship could continue, the decision to go to Denver when I was clearly ambivalent is deserving of rebuke. I could have discussed our relationship earlier. To initiate the rupture I became convinced was inevitable was going to be the most difficult thing I had ever done; it proved to be so. I had cared deeply, as had she. I am gratified that we have maintained contact. I am further gratified she is happily married. I departed Denver and went to the home in Rifle mother shared with Lefty, planning to spend several weeks. It was comforting to see that mother was receiving the kindness she deserved from a caring human. This unplanned interlude was a welcome respite before heading to Iowa. It would, unfortunately, be only a short while before mother's cancer diagnosis.

⋅⋅⋅

MY FIRST decade of employment in Iowa City, beginning in 1981, was characterized, in the main, by clinical duties and teaching. These related to residency and medical student training (staffing clinics, assisting and teaching in the operating room and on the labor and delivery suite, and general supervision when periodically assigned the obstetrical or gynecological service), as well as night call rotated among the staff. The work also included expansion of the Prenatal Diagnosis Clinic into the Fetal Diagnosis and Treatment Unit and organizing a statewide program to offer screening, by means of maternal blood tests, to pregnant women. The result of this testing could indicate an increased risk she would be carrying a fetus with a chromosome disorder such as Down syndrome or a fetus with an error in development such as a neural tube defect (opening in the spine). The vision and persistence of Dr. James Hanson facilitated the structure for optimal pregnancy screening protocols applied across the state, as well as for screening newborns for genetic diseases amenable to treatment before irreparable damage or death occurred. All of this was developed within a public health perspective and became a model for other states or regions.

A key figure who epitomized the strength of these programs was Dr. Stanton Berberich, long-time director of the central laboratory. He won the George Cunningham Visionary Award in newborn screening from the Association of Public Health Laboratories for implementing significant improvements which "demonstrated model practices for other newborn screening programs. He has been credited with improving timeliness of newborn screening in Iowa by establishing a courier system that operates daily and on holidays. He also established a night shift in the newborn screening laboratory to eliminate delays in screening." He implemented these changes to avoid deaths or serious disabilities were there to be delays in diagnosing infants with serious metabolic diseases. When Katrina struck New Orleans and incapacitated that program's ability to perform newborn screening tests, the blood samples were sent to the Iowa screening laboratory. This laboratory now performs the newborn screening tests for South Dakota, North Dakota, and Alaska.

Another entity integral to our work was the chromosome laboratory. For the duration of my employment, Dr. Shiva Patil and his lab staff expertly performed the chromosome evaluation from cells extracted from the fluids we sent him, most commonly amniotic fluid surrounding the fetus. I was privileged to have delivered the two children of Shiva and his wife Irene. Their daughter now practices Ob/Gyn. We have remained fast friends.

Dr. Hanson was preceded in his leadership role at Iowa by Dr. Johannes (Hans) Zellweger, who was recruited to the Department of Pediatrics in 1959. He was among the small cadre of physicians who had sought training in the nascent field of genetics. Prior to this training Dr. Zellweger worked for two years with Dr. Albert Schweitzer in Africa, giving serious consideration to devoting his life to this mission until tuberculosis forced him to relocate to Switzerland, the country of his birth. While serving as a member of the Swiss ski patrol, he assisted immigrants fleeing Nazi Germany. He became, for a time, head of the Department of Pediatrics at American University in Beirut. He identified children with a specific collection of abnormalities that became known as Zellweger syndrome. Dr. Hanson accelerated the efforts made by Dr. Zellweger, establishing Iowa as a state with a widely respected presence in birth defects surveillance, newborn screening, as mentioned, and human genomic studies, including the discovery of genes causing or predisposing to disease.

Dr. Zellweger was kind and caring but was "old school" in some of his approaches to patient problems. On at least two occasions he phoned me to discuss patients of his, both similar. In heavily accented diction he would describe a mentally challenged teenager, unable to care for herself and frightened and confused by monthly periods. "Roger," he would earnestly implore, "you can help her if you do a hysterectomy." I would patiently explain that I sympathized, but that legal counsel and ethical considerations (lack of ability to give informed consent and others) would not allow me to do so. I suggested other alternatives for his patient. He would softly grumble and conclude the conversation.

Though he did not understand nor agree with these restrictions, he had a deeply considered, independent moral code. As he related in a letter to those close to him toward the end of his life, he felt it was an obligation to not burden others by old age and mental and physical infirmity. At age 80 he took his life. According to those who knew him well, he was not depressed. He acknowledged he had lived a rich and full life. His affairs were attended to. He even left a check to cover emergency vehicle transportation to the medical school where he had willed his body to science. We cannot know whether he fully considered the grief this act would cause his family and friends.

As the decade of the 1980s progressed, those in our group caring for high-risk pregnancies became more involved in the prospect of treating fetuses for a number of different disorders. This was made possible by improved means to "see" or image a fetus, primarily by ultrasound, but also by other technologies such as magnetic resonance imaging or MRI,[46] and to partner with laboratory personnel to quickly diagnose and monitor treatment of fetuses, particularly those with anemia. Whereas fetal surgery for several disorders remains controversial, treatment of fetal anemia with blood transfusions has yielded gratifying results. There are numerous causes for fetal anemia, the most frequent being Rh disease, Rh referring to a protein carried on the membrane of the red blood cell (RBC; the oxygen carrying cell). Most people are Rh+, meaning their RBCs carry this protein as an antigen which can be attacked by an antibody. If an Rh- woman is carrying a fetus with this antigen (Rh+), some of these Rh+ fetal RBCs can gain access to the maternal circulation at the time of delivery. The maternal immune system will then recognize these cells as "foreign" because they carry a protein her system has not "seen" before. Her immune response may be the production of antibodies which can break down RBCs with this Rh protein. In any subsequent pregnancy in which she is carrying an Rh+ fetus, that fetus is at risk for anemia caused by maternal antibodies crossing the placenta and attacking RBCs of her fetus.

As a resident I remember several cases of severe fetal anemia causing fetal heart failure, resulting in death of the fetus. When Dr. Carl Weiner joined the faculty at Iowa, he developed an aggressive research and treatment program directed at fetal anemia, in which some of us actively participated over a number of years. We had earlier demonstrated a means to improve the safety of amniocentesis using thin needles and ultrasound guidance of the needle into the amniotic fluid.[47] This technique allowed needle insertion into the vein of the umbilical cord carrying blood into the fetal circulation, thereby allowing evaluation of the fetal blood count and transfusion, sometimes repeatedly over the course of a pregnancy, with healthy outcomes.[48,49]

During this decade I tried to remain involved in research at a more basic level, if only sporadically. Utilizing similar techniques developed for amniocentesis and fetal intrauterine transfusions, I collaborated with a group anticipating that gene therapy may become a future approach with applicability for fetuses. Were this to be the case, the most promising means to accomplish this would likely be delivery of the gene to a specific organ, and the most effective delivery vehicle would be viruses. With this strategy in mind, we were able to direct a small volume of virus carrying a known gene into the livers of fetal rabbits.[50] Subsequent studies in mice with defined disorders have shown the efficacy of this approach.[51]

These studies, and many others with which our group became involved, fell within the framework of an incipient network which got its start in 1982, and was formalized as the International Fetal Medicine and Surgery Society (IFMSS) in 1983. Presentations at yearly meetings included animal studies and evaluation and treatment of human fetuses. All submissions to the meeting were heard, and the open discussions were lively. The pediatric surgeon in our group, Dr. Kevin Pringle, was interested in diaphragmatic hernia, a defect in which a hole or opening in the dome-shaped muscle in the upper abdomen which aids breathing, the diaphragm, allows fetal bowel to escape into the chest and prevent proper development of the lungs, often leading to death shortly after birth despite surgery. His research involved a fetal sheep model of diaphragmatic hernia. His sheep came from a local farm at a modest cost. Nonetheless, his research budget was stretched thin and, as he was from New Zealand, the land of plentiful sheep, he decided to relocate to his native country. He has been an active participant in IFMSS since the beginning, including serving as president of the group and has hosted the annual meeting in New Zealand on two occasions.

Diaphragmatic hernia and fetal neural tube defects or openings in the spine were two leading candidates for operating on a fetus before birth. There were multiple challenges, but also promise within this field. Will fetuses with a neural tube defect, for example, have an improved long-term outcome—less paralysis below the opening, less difficulty with bowel and bladder function, greater chance to ambulate, less need for shunting to relieve a buildup of fluid in the brain (hydrocephalus)? Will the procedure justify the risks to the mother, and hence her fetus, of premature labor, rupture of the membranes surrounding her fetus, and others? The discussions about these and other issues were often passionate, and many are not settled. The aims of IFMSS were presentation of good studies and healthy debate to help answer these conundrums.

In the early days of attempts to treat fetuses, an ultrasound in our unit revealed a fetus with hydrocephalus, an excess of fluid in the ventricles, the spaces in the brain containing the cerebrospinal fluid. When a fetal abnormality is detected, counseling includes the offer to examine the fetal chromosome constitution via a procedure such as amniocentesis to assess whether the abnormality(ies) may be due to too much or too little chromosome material.[52] This was done, revealing a chromosomally normal male.

A group at the University of Colorado Medical School offered a procedure called shunting, the insertion of a tube into one of the ventricles of the fetus to shunt excess fluid into the amniotic fluid surrounding the fetus.[53] The goal for this treatment was to prevent ongoing damage to the developing brain from increasing pressure. The woman elected to go to Colorado and discuss her options with the Denver team. Ultimately, she chose to have the procedure performed and, by providing informed consent, accepted the risks to herself and her fetus. Several of us went to Denver and observed the successful placement of the catheter into the fetal ventricle under ultrasound guidance, performed at 22 weeks of gestation (a full-term pregnancy is 40 weeks). Multiple television stations were represented in a crowded room when the physicians provided details to the press following the procedure. The pregnancy progressed uneventfully until premature labor at 28 weeks resulted in delivery of a child with the catheter protruding from his skull. He ultimately did well following treatment for prematurity and placement of a permanent shunt. It was determined he had a "simple" blockage in a canal, preventing the normal flow of cerebrospinal fluid.

Though knowledge of birth defect causation, evaluative tools, and techniques to treat fetuses have improved considerably since this episode, it can still be difficult to select fetuses for these invasive procedures wherein the balance of risks and benefits may not be readily apparent. To cite the example of hydrocephalus, we looked in depth at our cases.[54] There was a great amount of heterogeneity, meaning there were many categorical causes, ranging from chromosomal abnormalities, certain viruses, disorders due to a single mutated gene, and those due to the combined effects of multiple genes (sometimes influenced by factors within the intrauterine environment). There was also a distressingly frequent "unknown" category. Within this latter category, hydrocephalus is often associated with multiple other birth defects. When an abnormality or collection of abnormalities is detected before birth, one must maintain an expansive view of the possibilities, particularly when fetal intervention is contemplated.

During this time the department Chair, Dr. Roy Pitkin, was not only editor of one of the two major journals in the field, but also of publications on specific topics. With his encouragement, this permitted a forum for me to summarize advances in the field of fetal surgery[55] and to guest edit a series of chapters on prenatal diagnosis,[56] including a contribution with Dr. Jeffrey Murray titled *Molecular Analyses of Genetic Disorders*.[57] I also began a close working relationship with the Reproductive Endocrine division of our department. When Dr. Craig Syrop initiated the in vitro fertilization (IVF) program, I helped him retrieve oocytes or eggs for fertilization in tissue culture dishes in the early days of the program. The IVF program has gained a deserved national reputation over the years, subsequently headed by Dr. Bradley van Voorhis. The critical laboratory aspects of IVF have been directed by Dr. Amy Sparks. Their team has conducted research over many years which has helped secure IVF on a more solid scientific and ethical foundation.[58] Dr. Sparks has kept the program on the cutting edge, incorporating new developments into the laboratory in a timely fashion such as preimplantation genetic diagnosis (PGD).[59] If a couple is at risk to have a child with a serious genetic disease, a single cell is removed from the embryos by Dr. Sparks following IVF and sent overnight to a laboratory specializing in making a genetic diagnosis from DNA of a single cell; only unaffected embryos are transferred to the uterus following PGD. I have had many interchanges with this group about the importance of genetics in their field.[60]

This early decade of mostly clinical work and teaching was fulfilling, but I had the sense that academic work would be enhanced if I could pursue more basic research. I had discussions with a colleague, Dr. Jeffrey Murray. His knowledge about this expanding world of molecular genetics was one factor which stirred a desire to become more involved in "hard core" science. Pursuing an MS in medical school and working in a laboratory in Seattle had provided only a glimpse of the personal intellectual benefit. I wanted to substantively learn the genetic technologies driving so many of the basic findings in medicine and biology. To effectively accomplish this would require a sabbatical year at another institution. Sabbaticals were allowed, even encouraged, if one could bring expertise back to the medical school not then existing, but they were competitive.

I had been reading about a series of technologies which would allow the inactivation of a single gene in mice; the parlance was "knocking out" the function of a gene such that the protein that gene specified or coded for was not made, producing a knockout (KO) mouse (murine) strain. Though mice and humans evolutionarily diverged from a common ancestor about 75 million years ago, there remains a high degree of commonality in the genetic structure of the two species. Therefore, if the hitherto unknown function of a gene is discerned by its elimination in mice, this has great relevance for understanding the function of that gene in humans. Also, if a mutated human gene is the cause of disease, a KO of that gene in mice often produces a model which reasonably replicates the human disease, allowing detailed studies and novel therapeutic attempts which could not be done in humans.[61]

Dr. Pitkin left Iowa City in 1988 to become department Chair at UCLA. His replacement was Dr. Jennifer Niebyl. When I discussed my plans with her, she was supportive. I next had to submit a proposal to the institutional office overseeing sabbaticals and secure a position in one of the few laboratories pursuing the work at this time, principally those of Dr. Mario Capecchi at the medical school in Salt Lake City and Dr. Oliver Smithies at the University of North Carolina Medical School in Chapel Hill. I called Dr. Capecchi and was surprised when it was he who answered. I stated my desire to spend a sabbatical year in his lab. Without apologies, he indicated his lab could not take on another individual. I thanked him. Fearful of another blunt rejection, I took a deep breath, phoned Dr. Smithies, and was passed through to him. He answered with a friendly, distinctly British accent. I repeated my rehearsed script and responded to a few of his questions. He indicated I should come to Chapel Hill to discuss this further. He offered an overnight stay in the house he shared with Dr. Nobuyo Maeda, his scientific colleague in their laboratory and future wife. Such generosity extended to someone in my circumstance is not the norm.

Dr. Smithies—I will call him Oliver—had a shock of curly grey hair. It did not take long to discern he was a modest, open man without pretensions. After a visit to the laboratory and an overnight with him and Dr. Maeda, they drove me to the airport. Their decision had not been announced. My background, particularly a lack of experience with basic molecular techniques, did not make me a particularly attractive candidate. But Dr. Smithies' approach to science was collaborative and sharing. He knew the value of KO technology to the scientific community and wanted it spread widely. It may also have helped that during dinner the conversation turned to flying, Oliver's avid hobby, allowing me to interject that I had done some flying in the Navy. He exited the car at the airport entrance, and as we shook hands he said the affirmative words I was hoping to hear; "Yes, I think this will work." The proposal I submitted for the sabbatical was approved, and within a few months I was in North Carolina.

That sabbatical year, ending the summer of 1990, was a superlative learning experience. Creating a KO murine line at that time was daunting, requiring success at all steps of this multi-stage, often multi-year experiment. The starting material for these experiments was murine embryonic stem (ES) cells, capable of becoming every cell in the body of an organism, in this case contributing to all the organs of a developing mouse, including gametes (eggs and sperm). These remarkable ES cells were isolated in 1981 by Sir Martin Evans in Great Britain.[62] When ES cells divide in a tissue culture dish, they form rounded colonies. I vividly recall an almost childlike sense of wonder when Dr. Maeda beckoned me to look at a colony under the microscope, one portion of which was beating in synchrony, the earliest vestige of a heart. Some intrinsic program had been initiated; a group of cells had spontaneously linked up, electrically coupled, and started down the cardiac pathway. I could imagine no starker demonstration that these cells are primed to create organs. This evidence of self-organization is one of the recurring themes in stem cell research and organismal development.

To accomplish a KO, a DNA "construct" is engineered in the laboratory which has homology (similar or same sequence) to the gene of interest. This construct is introduced into ES cells and "seeks out" the area of homology on the DNA in the nucleus. If this happens, the construct DNA can replace the native DNA sequence through the process of homologous recombination. This is the same process that occurs when ova and sperm are made (meiosis). During meiosis the chromosomes pair off and exchange homologous portions of DNA along their lengths. If the construct DNA is engineered properly, the gene will be inactivated following homologous recombination. When this is accomplished, these genetically modified ES cells are injected into early-stage organisms (blastocysts) where they can contribute to all cell populations, including gametes. The blastocysts are then transferred to the reproductive tracts of recipient females for further gestation. The desired alteration of sperm cells of subsequently born pups can lead, following appropriate breeding trials, to mice which do not express or produce the protein of interest; hence, a KO murine line.

Oliver's interest in homologous recombination derived from his desire to help cure disease, specifically to correct genetic diseases by this form of gene therapy, targeted replacement of a disease-causing gene by a normal copy. It was known that homologous recombination could occur in yeast, but it was far from certain, at the time he was conducting these studies, that this could be accomplished in mammals. He set his sights on sickle cell anemia. The goals he established were, for the time, ambitious and risky. Graduate students, whose future careers depend upon research success, shunned the opportunity to work on this project initially, so Oliver performed the research planning and much of the bench work, revealing that he could successfully introduce an engineered piece of DNA into the sickle cell gene by homologous recombination in cultured mammalian cells.[63] He and colleagues later showed they could correct the gene causing sickle cell disease by replacement with the normal gene in mammalian cells.[64] These experiments were a prelude to his murine gene targeting work.

It was planned that I would conduct research under Dr. Maeda's guidance. Her expertise was the genetics of atherosclerotic heart disease. We had success with a gene which was fortunately very susceptible to targeted replacement, apolipoprotein A-1, ultimately producing a murine model with reduced levels of cholesterol.[65] Without her help and that of many lab mates, this project would have foundered. So many aspects of this year were gratifying. The experiment was successful in the time I was allotted. While doing this work, I was able to perform many of the extant molecular biological techniques at the bench. Absorption in this science was thoroughly engrossing, involving so many areas of personal interest, including stem cell biology, basic genetics, and reproductive biology. The broad sweep of this experience proved invaluable when I transferred this technology back to Iowa.

In addition to the intellectual stimulation of this scientific environment, Oliver's love of flying was an unanticipated bonus. He enjoyed taking students in his lab on flights around Chapel Hill in his motorized glider. When he went to meetings or to give talks in the United States, he flew his slighter larger Cessna 180. But he enjoyed gliding and could do so without needing another plane to tow him to altitude before release. He could take off unaided, and when at a designated altitude could turn off the motor, flatten the prop, and glide. He was a keen student of flying. I marveled at how relaxed he was while gliding, searching for vortices to gain altitude, watching for birds doing the same, thereby revealing these updrafts.

Oliver sensed I wanted to fly with him any time he indicated. Not infrequently, while I was working at the bench, he would appear around a corner, smile, and raise his eyebrows in an inquiring gesture; his invitation to go flying. I would wrap up as quickly as possible. He knew from our previous conversations that I had taken flying lessons in the Navy, though had not obtained a pilot's license. On an early flight he indicated he was an instructor, and would I like to complete this goal with him? Of course I would. Oliver was a natural teacher and a pleasant person to be with. In my presence, and no doubt with others, he was loquacious, the subjects usually confined to science and flying. So, about mid-way into the year I began lessons with him in his motorized glider. These were progressing well. I had soloed during the lessons in the Navy, so was confident this step would come quickly. I had not thought ahead to the time I would apply for a permanent license and the form would ask about my health, including depression. I had truthfully answered this question only one time—filling out the forms for employment at the University of Iowa. This admission was treated respectfully and did not cause a reconsideration of my status.

I cherished these times with Oliver, though they were not to last. I was piloting the aircraft with Oliver alongside. The plan was to land on a small grass strip near the town of Keener. The landing was uneventful. The long wings of the plane cleared the un-mowed portion of grass flanking the strip, but not by much. I turned the plane in preparation for takeoff. When just airborne the plane abruptly spun one hundred eighty degrees and landed hard on the runway. We were uninjured, but the undercarriage was badly damaged. In retrospect, the only plausible cause of this mishap was a wing tip dipping into the thick grass, sending the plane into the spin. My flying days were over. I have not re-engaged with the hobby, probably for the best. When I flew solo in the Navy, I never became confident or comfortable, though with more experience this was certainly a longed-for possibility. Oliver told me on several occasions that his becoming a confident pilot had translated into confidence in other spheres of his life. It was somehow comforting to know that this man of such accomplishment could ever have lacked confidence.

When the sabbatical year ended, I returned to many of my prior responsibilities. Additionally, I joined a three-person group providing "private" deliveries; in reality, most of the patients were quite accepting of delivery by a resident with our close supervision. The top priority upon returning was establishment of a laboratory to transfer the procedures learned in Chapel Hill, including working closely with animal care personnel to maintain a pathogen-free (sterile) environment for the mice. As was the case for all human studies, local Institutional Review Boards required that research with animals, including mice, be conducted under rigorous standards. I served for a time on the committee overseeing animal research and can verify this committee closely monitored adherence to strict standards to avoid unnecessary risk and pain.

In addition to the animal care facility, I would also need collaborators whose area of expertise would benefit from this technology. It was soon apparent there were many who had this need. The medical school subsidized core facilities to aid investigators, and, after multiple discussions, the research administration designated our facility a core, the Gene Targeting Core Facility, and supplied start-up funds. Within several years another significant asset, Dr. Baoli Yang, joined the laboratory. He was a trainee in Oliver's laboratory, as was his wife, who was accepted into our Ob/Gyn residency.

Dr. Niebyl was also helpful. Her history of advancement in a field dominated by men throughout most of her career is exceptional. She led in an even-handed manner and maintained equanimity in the face of difficult obstacles. She first became a nurse on advice of her parents, who counseled that the rigors of medicine would be too much for a woman. Nonetheless, she went to medical school, then completed a Fellowship in maternal fetal medicine (high risk pregnancies) following residency. She has organized and published important studies and become an author of multi-authored textbooks in general Ob/Gyn and her chosen subspecialty. When she accepted the offer as Chair at Iowa, a position she held for 21 years, she was only the fourth woman to lead a department of Ob/Gyn in this country. In a series in one of the two top-tier journals in our field, she was designated one of the Giants in Obstetrics and Gynecology.[66] Perhaps this recognition will render that appellation, Giant, more gender-neutral?

Several months after returning I received a phone call from Oliver. He was flying to Iowa City: could I pick him up for an overnight in my house? Then he explained his reason for coming. He had belonged to a flying club in Madison when he was on faculty at the University of Wisconsin. For many years the club organized a yearly, members-only, quirky flying contest in Keokuk, a small Iowa town at the extreme southeast corner on the Mississippi River, at the invitation of a local resident and friend of many club members. That evening in Iowa City I inquired if he would talk informally with the Medical Genetics faculty and staff the following day. It was easy to ask; I knew he would readily consent. We then flew to Keokuk and checked into a motel. That night he explained the contest guidelines. Over breakfast the triangular route to be flown for this competition would be revealed. These morning instructions called for participants to depart Keokuk, fly to Macomb and Galesburg in Illinois, then back to Keokuk. The pilot who had most closely calculated fuel consumption and estimated time to land back at Keokuk would be declared winner. After Oliver scribbled his calculations on a piece of paper we left. My assigned task was to record some of the relevant numbers. The varieties and vintages of aircraft in the contest were astonishing. The pilot-to-pilot chatter among these long-time buddies, the friendly belittlement of other nearby contestants in the air, belied a deep camaraderie. One of the planes was piloted by Field Morey, the person who taught Oliver to fly. I was later to learn that the two of them flew across the Atlantic in a Cessna 210. During the leg from Goose Bay, Labrador to Reykjavik, Iceland they set a speed record for that class of aircraft that stood for 20 years. Alas, for all his expertise, Oliver did not place on that day in Keokuk.

In addition to coming to Iowa City to participate in the Keokuk festivities, Oliver was invited to the medical school on two further occasions. He was a well-known and respected scientist, asked to give many lectures nationally and internationally. He generously accepted as many of these invitations as he could manage. In 2002 he participated in A Celebration of Academic Medicine at Iowa and gave two talks to large and appreciative audiences. The first was titled, "Fifty Years at the Lab Bench as a Biomedical Scientist," and the second was, "My Mouse Solutions to Human Problems." He was wearing one of the few sweaters he rotated, speaking in his beguiling accent, revealing his way of doing science which was increasingly deviating from the trend fostered by Big Science—data mining the results of large, multi-center collaborative projects, often, as he decried, not driven by hypotheses. He devised experiments, performed them at the bench, sometimes making equipment he needed but not available, filling notebooks with reams of entries on his results and his thoughts about them, and plans for tomorrow's or future experiments. These notebooks, with their insights into the workings of Oliver's mind, have been archived by the University of North Carolina.

The third talk he gave in Iowa City was at the invitation of graduate students, a group favored by him, accepting at a time when he was even more besieged by invitations. This spike in requests was occasioned by a glorious achievement; in 2007 he was recipient of the Nobel Prize in Medicine or Physiology, along with co-recipients Dr. Mario Capecchi and Sir Martin Evans. When I heard this, I had a real sense of the ceremony to come. Years earlier I was taken to the Orchestra Hall in Stockholm, site of the evening's tributes. I could picture Oliver with his beaming smile, paying homage to his fellow scientists, former students and trainees, and to the science of which he was such a creative practitioner.

As the Nobel attested, Oliver was always striving to push boundaries. He did so in science as well as in flying. I have mentioned his transatlantic flight with Field Morey. Oliver also desired to attain the Diamond Award in gliding, an altitude goal. He first went to a chamber complex in Milwaukee where he could be decompressed to the equivalent of 30,000 feet of altitude. As a part of this drill, he was required to remove his oxygen mask for 90 seconds at that altitude to experience the mental effects of hypoxia (low oxygen), not unlike a state of being inebriated. Following this he went to a glider port near Denver. When the west winds come over the mountains, vortices can be generated at high altitude. He selected a winter day with favorable gliding conditions, was towed to 14,000 feet and released, and then climbed to 30,800, a gain of 16,800 feet. These figures allowed Oliver to attain the Diamond designation. The goals he established were self-motivated. He was not conflicted by external pressure. In my interactions with him he displayed an ease and serenity we rarely associate with hard-charging individuals pursuing goals established by others.

The sabbatical Oliver allowed me led to the most satisfying aspect of my employment, a subsequent 20-year period of association and collaboration with outstanding investigators, including two who were recipients of Howard Hughes Medical Institute funds, Drs. Kevin Campbell and Michael Welsh. When Howard Hughes died, the fortune of this eccentric billionaire was set aside to fund only the most deserving scientists, allowing them independence in their use of these funds, subject to periodic review. Dr. Campbell's research focused primarily on skeletal muscle, principally the degeneration associated with muscular dystrophies. There are many forms of muscular dystrophy caused by mutations in single genes; the most common is Duchenne muscular dystrophy, affecting only males. The goal was to produce KO mice which would hopefully model their human counterparts with sufficient fidelity to understand how the gene disruption causes muscle disease in humans, which may point toward specific therapies. Many instructive models resulted from this work. As an example, after a specific type of muscular dystrophy KO had been created,[67] a therapy with future potential to help humans with this disease was reported.[68]

As KO technology became more sophisticated, it was possible to inactivate the function of a gene in a specific tissue, the remainder of the tissues retaining an intact copy of the gene of interest. When we inactivated a protein intimately involved with skeletal muscle function, dystroglycan, this caused early demise of the embryos.[69] However, when this protein was absent only in brain tissue, the mice lived but their brains developed abnormally, displaying features which often accompany congenital (born with) varieties of muscular dystrophy.[70] This study reveals an important, commonly recognized feature of genes; they can be expressed in multiple tissues, a characteristic referred to as pleiotropy.

Dr. Campbell had a collaborator in Upsala, Sweden, the home of Carl Linnaeus, the taxonomist who specified a system for the classification of organisms. The collaborator had requested a meeting to discuss aspects of their joint research. Dr. Campbell was unable to go, so asked if I would fill in for him. Toward the end of our time together, the collaborator asked if I would like a tour of the Karolinska Institute in Stockholm—a facility well-known for medical care and research. The facility is also home to the Nobel Assembly which, in turn, chooses Nobel Prize awardees. During the tour the Karolinska scientist showed me the interior of Orchestra Hall where, as previously mentioned, Nobel recipients receive their prizes in elaborately staged performances. I only found out later that my guide was one of the professors from the various disciplines within the Karolinska Institute who choose the Nobel awardees.

While in Sweden I also visited the famed Vasa Museum in Stockholm which houses this magnificent vessel. The *Vasa* was a ship improperly balanced, and it ingloriously sank on its maiden voyage in 1628 as it sailed out to sea to battle Poland, in sight of large crowds lining the banks. It lay on the bottom until 1921 when salvage crews dredged beneath the ship, attached cables, and raised this now expertly conserved ship, among the most significant ever excavated.

In addition to production of murine models of muscular dystrophy, I became involved in another area of research, the study of ion channels which are a major contributor to disease.[71] Ion channels ferry charged (negative or positive) ions like chloride, sodium, and potassium into and out of cells. One of our experiments highlighted the importance of one such channel for the structure of an area of the brain called the hippocampus, critical for memory formation. When one of numerous chloride channels was inactivated, the hippocampus completely degenerated![72] Ion channels were the research focus of another distinguished investigator at the medical school, Dr. Michael Welsh, previously mentioned. It was his group that determined that cystic fibrosis (CF), a disease in which secretions, particularly lung secretions, become thick and viscous, was due to a defect in yet another chloride channel.[73] In humans many organs are affected by CF, but it is the lung pathology which is most concerning and most frequently causes death. A bright and talented postdoctoral student in Oliver's laboratory, Dr. Beverly Koller, worked diligently for years (as did other groups) to KO this chloride channel to produce murine CF. I witnessed the diligence required to finally succeed.[74]

CF is caused by over 1,000 distinct mutations. This disease exemplifies the progress made in many genetic disorders, from clinical identification of the disease to discovery of the causative gene and its function in the cell. Attempts were initially made to treat CF with gene therapy. For this disease, these efforts have been supplanted by the design of drugs which have ameliorated the symptoms and increased life span for most individuals with CF. Michael Welsh has been a major figure in this long, difficult saga.[75]

Not all murine models of single gene disorders will faithfully replicate their human counterparts. Unfortunately, although the CF mice had gastrointestinal pathology and other manifestations which can affect humans, the mice did not have lung involvement. Therefore, Dr. Welsh and colleagues turned to the pig. By utilizing cutting-edge techniques, they were able to create pigs with CF (a porcine model), including the devastating lung disease.[76] These techniques included a step to change the normal pig CF gene to a mutated version via gene targeting. The nuclei of the correctly targeted cells were removed and inserted into porcine ova from which the nuclei were removed. This and the steps which followed were those which produced the first cloned mammal, the sheep named Dolly. The great value of these models, murine, porcine, and many others, is that they allow therapies to be tested, studies impermissible in humans. Dr. Welsh and his co-investigators showed, in a preliminary way, that the normal CF gene, carried by a viral vector and delivered to the airways of CF pigs, could partially correct the lung pathology.[77]

Dr. Welsh was also involved with other channels which influence health, including a large family of sodium channel genes comprised of subunits. We collaborated on the KO of one of these subunits of the murine epithelial sodium channel which resulted in death shortly after birth.[78] However, it was the inactivation of another channel related to the sodium channel family, an acid sensing channel (ASIC1a), activated by a fall in pH, which Drs. Welsh and John Wemmie worked on with another group.[79] This KO exposed a previously unexplored aspect of brain function with implications for anxiety and depression.[80] Sophisticated studies have revealed that many models of genetically altered mice can display scientifically tractable behaviors related to fear processing in humans. Acid sensing in the amygdala, a key brain region for coordinating behaviors related to fear, has been recognized as an important newer insight by one of the noted investigators in this field, Joseph LeDoux.[81]

The murine stem cell work our core laboratory was conducting was consuming and gratifying. However, when it became apparent that cells from mice and humans, long thought to be fixed in their mature or fully differentiated identity, were proven to be plastic or changeable, this commanded the attention of the scientific community. Japanese investigators, led by Dr. Shinya Yamanaka, first showed that fibroblasts, cells isolated from the skin of mice, were capable of a remarkable transformation. When these cells were infected with viruses carrying one of four genes which are key to maintaining cells in an undifferentiated state, a small percent of these fibro-blasts reversed their previous differentiation pathway; they dedifferentiated and became stem cells,[82] with properties comparable to the embryonic stem cells which had previously been isolated from murine embryos.

The term applied to these cells is induced pluripotent stem cells or iPSCs. One year after murine iPSCs were derived, human fibroblasts were reverted to iPSCs by a procedure similar to that for creating murine iPSCs,[83,84] showing properties like those possessed by ES cells isolated from both murine and human embryos.[85] ES cells have been isolated from human embryos donated by couples undergoing IVF who have completed their childbearing goals. This method of obtaining ES cells is ethically troubling to many. Stem cells produced from fibroblasts do not carry these ethical implications. Basic immunology provides another distinct iPSC advantage when stem cell therapy is contemplated. If a patient donates his/her cells for conversion to iPSCs destined for treatment—after the appropriate protocol to differentiate them into therapeutic cells—these cells will be accepted as one's "own." The demonstration that adult cells were so plastic they could be converted to embryonic stem cells led to a Nobel Prize for Dr. Yamanaka only six years after his original publication, an historically short time between a scientific breakthrough and the Nobel.

Dr. Campbell, meanwhile, continued to make progress on many fronts in the quest to understand the mechanistic details underlying many forms of muscular dystrophy. This knowledge is requisite for the development of specific, targeted treatments. In 2005, under his leadership, the University of Iowa Paul D. Wellstone Muscular Dystrophy Cooperative Center was established, the funds administered through a branch of the NIH. Paul Wellstone was a feisty Democratic senator from Minnesota who tragically died in a small plane crash in 2002. Dr. Campbell received a renewal of funds for this Center in 2015 to continue research on finding treatments for muscular dystrophies.

It was the combination of the iPSC work of Dr. Yamanaka and others and funding of the Wellstone Center that led to me to switch from murine gene targeting to iPSC work. The leadership of the Gene Targeting Core Facility had previously been transferred to the very capable Dr. Yang. I received modest funds from the Wellstone grant to conduct research and from the university to help fund a laboratory devoted to this work. My project was predicated on converting fibroblasts from patients with a variety of muscular dystrophies into iPSCs, and then differentiating these iPSC lines into muscle tissue, with the goal of determining the mechanisms by which the dystrophic or degenerative process occurred. The fibroblasts had previously been isolated from skin biopsies of consenting patients by Dr. Steven Moore, co-director of the Wellstone Center. Satisfactory progress was being made when I decided to retire in 2010.

Another area of intense investigation is the production of three-dimensional derivatives of iPSCs called organoids. In contrast to the attempt to derive a single cell type in the lab such as dopamine-producing neurons to treat Parkinson disease, organoids are small bits of a specific tissue. The culture conditions are different for each tissue (growth factors, etc.), simulating the stages of development of that tissue. Organoids of brain[86] and many other tissues have been coaxed from normal iPSCs and from patient-derived iPSCs, patients with disorders of brain structure and/or function. The potential to understand disease processes utilizing organoids is vast. I was intrigued when trophoblast organoids, with features of early placentas, were grown in culture.[87] There is much to be learned about the placenta, the interface between mother and her fetus, an organ often dysfunctional in many disorders of pregnancy and a key organ preventing immune rejection of the fetus.

As I approached the age of retirement, I frequently reflected that I had, indeed, been fortunate in career choices and the leaders I had. Though my Fellowship training was in Medical Genetics, I became a member of the maternal fetal medicine (MFM) division. The MFM division directors, Carl Weiner, previously mentioned for his fetal transfusion expertise, and his successor, Dr. Jerome Yankowitz (board certified in both MFM *and* medical genetics) set lofty goals for the Fetal Diagnosis and Treatment Unit. Both went on to become Chairs of Departments of OB/Gyn at other institutions.

Though negative intrusive thoughts laced with reproach were still commonly inserted into ongoing brain activity, they became somewhat less frequent and "softer" than in the past. Regular exercise, even when motivation was flagging, has been a significant help over the years. I was also fortunate that for the decades spanning Fellowship training to the present, I have had mutually reinforcing relationships. Of many who have been friends and aided me in many ways, two people have been considerable helpmates.

When their parents were divorcing, Stanley Grant and her brother were deposited at their grandparent's home when she was eight months old. They were raised with love, but many privations. As a nurse genetic counselor, she "ran" our Fetal Diagnosis and Therapy Clinic, helping me and my colleagues in numerous ways with organization and sensitive patient care. She also applied these skills to our statewide Maternal Serum Pregnancy Screening Program. I have known S. Derrickson Moore since the beginning of my Fellowship. She has pursued many worthwhile goals as a journalist and concerned citizen and has been a fount of wisdom.

Before turning to events post-retirement, more commentary about other advances in the era of molecular biology is warranted. Another collaborator recruited to Iowa by Dr. Hanson was Dr. Jeffrey Murray, previously mentioned. He is a past president of the 9,000 member American Society of Human Genetics. His productive laboratory was involved in coordinating other groups of scientists conducting large genomic studies here and abroad to identify genes or regions of the genome predisposing to illness. He was equally known for moral suasion regarding patient advocacy, international health, social and health policy, and the immense ethical and legal issues raised by the field of genetics. He was a trainee in medical genetics in the Seattle program after I left. While there, he completed a study I had been associated with.[88] We have collaborated on several subsequent projects, including studies to discriminate regions of the genome which predispose to preeclampsia,[89, 90] a serious disorder of pregnancy consisting of the triad of maternal hypertension, protein in the urine, and accumulation of fluid (edema).

The possibility of gaining knowledge in the field of genetics was accelerated when the human genome was sequenced. This accomplishment was fostered by the establishment of human genome centers, initially two in the U.S. and one in France. Iowa hosted one of these, the Cooperative Human Linkage Center (CHLC), directed by Jeff and Dr. Val Sheffield. One of the charges for this center was to establish genetic markers along the lengths of the 23 pairs of human chromosomes.[91] These markers facilitated discovery of disease-causing genes and greatly aided the studies which led to the eventual sequencing of the human genome. I recall Dr. Francis Collins, NIH Director and leader of the NIH sequencing effort, coming to the medical school to acknowledge (celebrate really) the CHLC's role. During his remarks, Dr.

Collins lauded the team for rarely achieved accomplishments with funded projects; coming in on time and under budget. Another noteworthy aspect of the CHLC was that it was the first project of its kind to include a medical ethicist, Iowa faculty member Dr. Robert Weir, among the investigators. This became a routine feature of large genomic studies headed by Jeff. He, the other scientists at Iowa I have mentioned, and many more have contributed to the large role Iowa has played in the genetics revolution.[92]

⁝⁝⁝

AS MUST be the case for many contemplating retirement, I was ambivalent. However, this emotion did not linger; within a week of retirement in 2010 I was back in Turkey. George Bass and his co-workers had spent the summer of 1960 excavating a Bronze Age shipwreck at Cape Gelidonya, referenced earlier. He contacted the surviving members of his 1960 crew to again assemble at Cape Gelidonya to celebrate the fiftieth anniversary of this first scientifically credible underwater excavation. He also planned an Institute of Nautical Archeology (INA) project to search for any remaining artifacts or fragments left on the seabed. Since his diving had been curtailed by a stroke, he assigned one of INA's Research Associates to direct the project; I would serve as physician.

Over the years I have perused the vast tome resulting from this initial excavation.[93] To assist this effort, George had recruited a talented group; skillful divers included Frédéric Dumas, Jacque Cousteau's chief diver, and Waldemar Illing from Germany; other underwater archeologists including Honor Frost; and his best friend Claude Duthuit, the grandson of the French painter Henri Matisse. Claude had the means to indulge his many passions, including diving and underwater archeology. The scholarly publication resulting from this project helped establish high academic standards for underwater archeology. Multiple other shipwrecks have been excavated and published by members of INA. The most significant one to date was another Bronze Age craft found at Uluburun, near Cape Gelidonya. It required 11 seasons of work at the site, the majority led by a protégé of George's, Cemal Pulak who grew up in Turkey. My return to Cape Gelidonya in 2010 provided the opportunity to know this dedicated scholar and his work.[94]

There were remaining artifacts which were recovered during the 2010 Cape Gelidonya project, but the excavation in 1960 under trying circumstances was remarkably thorough. I dove to the wreck site several times, but I was the piker of the group, having not participated in this activity since 1974. The current was often strong and bothersome. Once, on descending, I inadvertently separated from the rope line extending from the dive barge to the wreck, was caught in the current, and when I broke surface was about 100 yards from the dive barge. When the three friends from the original excavation, George, Claude Duthuit, and Waldemar Illing, wanted to make a commemorative dive, I was conflicted. George had recovered significant function lost when he had the stroke, but concern remained. Also, before the proposed dive, Claude Duthuit had informed me he had coronary bypass surgery, adding it had been performed by Dr. Denton Cooley, Baylor College of Medicine surgeon. (I refrained from telling him I had been a student on his service decades earlier.) Despite the red flags, I was powerless to disallow this dive. It was all hands-on deck. I had the fully stocked medicine cabinet close at hand. The recompression chamber was, as always, on site. Fortunately, the current was low on this morning, and all went well, though these intrepid divers were spent at the conclusion of the dive.

In addition to serving on the board of INA, I have also been a member of this organization's Archeological Committee whose function is to review project proposals and fund the worthiest of them from monies donated to INA. Membership on National Institutes of Health study sections, convened to evaluate submitted molecular biology research proposals and disperse funds, had prepared me well for this task. For many years the annual meeting of the Archeological Committee was held in College Station, Texas, the home of George and Ann Bass. I stayed at their home in a room lined with hundreds of operas in DVD format, George's favored diversion. He had a sophisticated knowledge of opera. On Friday nights he invited students to his home for pizza and opera, sparsely attended initially, but as enthusiasm grew so did the attendance. My knowledge about George and Ann and their extended families increased during our conversations, but greatly expanded when George shared his meticulously researched family history of their forebears.

From the beginning in 1960, George's career continued an impressive trajectory of significant excavations in the Mediterranean, scholarly publications, National Geographic articles, lectures, and books for lay audiences.[95,96] His fraternity of land-based archeologists recognized his pioneering contributions to the field.[97] George was awarded a National Medal of Science by President George W. Bush. Many other awards were bestowed; a significant acknowledgment of his scholarship and keen intellect was certified in a Time magazine special edition titled *Great Scientists: The Geniuses, Eccentrics, and Visionaries Who Transformed Our World.*[98] In this publication he was placed among those we commonly associate with superior intelligence and accomplishment; Einstein, Newton, Marie Curie, Freud, and others. We should be appropriately cautious of lists such as this. However, we are a list-making species, and it is in that spirit that I acknowledge George's mental prowess.

Through INA I encountered another scientist with an irrepressible personality, Robert Ballard, best known for his discovery of the *Titanic*, though he had a long history of ocean exploration in and out of the Navy. It was the Navy which funded his discovery of the *Titanic*, kept secret at the time because his primary mission was to find two submarines which had sunk in the North Atlantic, the *Thresher* and the *Scorpion*. For a time, Dr. Ballard was on the board of INA, and in 2010 he hosted the annual board meeting at the University of Rhode Island where he was Director of the Center for Ocean Exploration in the Graduate School of Oceanography. We toured his facility with its numerous panels displaying, in real time, the images sent back to the Center from the remotely operated vehicle deployed from his research vessel via a high bandwidth satellite link. On our tour he joked that the relationships he had established with biologists and archeologists meant that he could send images of an unfamiliar deep-sea creature or an archeological finding to these experts, any hour of the day, to determine their significance.

As the meeting was ending, he announced he was driving to Boston, but could drop anyone off at the Providence airport on the way. I was the only person who could benefit from this offer. It struck me I might have to carry some of the conversation on the ride. He could not possibly want to again recount the *Titanic* story. His long history of underwater exploration, particularly with the little workhorse submersible, *Alvin*, was of interest to me. Perhaps we could discourse on *Alvin* and other submersibles. My worry about contribution to a topic, or lack thereof, was unfounded. This voluble man talked throughout the trip about his Center, future leadership changes he envisioned, and speculation about the future of his field. He was flying to

Houston for a fundraiser. As he was dropping me off, I mused to myself that his enthusiasm, coupled with his expertise and reputation, would almost certainly guarantee this Houston trip would be a successful outing.

George and Dr. Ballard were friends, each respecting the other's work. INA collaborated on one project in the Black Sea where Dr. Ballard was concentrating a portion of his deep-water exploration. Several years after this collaboration George was offered, and seized upon, the opportunity to descend to the *Titanic* in a Russian submersible with Russian pilots, at the time the only conveyance to the shipwreck. Similarly, for years the only means to convey supplies and personnel to the International Space Station was a Russian spacecraft.

After retirement I joined a well-established group of health care providers representing the Community Health Initiative on one of their trips to the beleaguered country of Haiti, still recovering from a devastating earthquake in 2010. One of the co-founders of this nonprofit was Dr. Chris Buresh, an Emergency Room physician on the faculty of the medical school in Iowa City. He was present for this trip, as he is for many of them. Care was provided to residents of several towns near the capital of Port-au-Prince who were able to get to the clinics from surrounding areas. The hard work, dedication, and vision of these volunteers were inspiring. The organization and their leaders have taken an expansive view of health, much needed when the root causes of poor health reflect broader needs. Over many years they have established a plastic recycling service in the capital, have arranged for latrines to be built, wells to be dug, funded a hydrogeologic survey to find sources of underground water, sponsored youth soccer games, and dispensed clean birthing kits for sanitary deliveries and to aid the newborn's breathing.

Several books helped me understand this country and the mission of medical groups volunteering in Haiti. Prior to 1804 France ruled the territory and profited from the efforts of slaves. In 1804 a slave rebellion successfully evicted the French and established the country of Haiti, the only time in history a slave uprising has led to this result.[99] Tracy Kidder has written a revealing book about Partners in Health providing medical care in Haiti and other countries, headed by their peripatetic leader, Dr. Paul Farmer.[100] Almost everything one hears or reads about Haiti is negative; the country seems in constant turmoil, but the situation is more nuanced. For me, this reality and common perception was offset by the people we encountered in the clinics. Despite their deprivation, the patients were dignified, resilient, and proud. Many elderly patients were carried by relatives or brought by donkey long distances over mountains to receive care.

As a result of this single experience in delivery of health care to under-served nations, I gained increased respect for Tim, my brother, who makes a yearly trip to Honduras to provide care to a severely needy population, sometimes accompanied by his wife Mary Ann, a Nurse Practitioner. For decades they have practiced in the same office, he as the only pediatrician in Ojai, California and the surrounding area. They are popular and respected members of the community. A float in one of the town parades was ridden by numerous children with the banner "Tim's Kids." He also works in a busy Emergency Room in Ventura, seeing patients of all ages. This has obviously required him to update and expand his knowledge base and skill sets to include seeing/treating adults, not a trivial undertaking. He has continued this very busy schedule well into his 70s. He and his wife have two sons.

Until I went to Haiti, I was unaware that Dr. Robert Hilgers, the oncol-ogist who skillfully and sensitively cared for Nancy, previously mentioned, has also devoted decades of service to the women of Haiti. Their rate of cervical cancer is many-fold higher than in the U.S. because of a lack of screening. Their cancers are also not usually detected until late in the course of the disease. Dr. Hilgers founded the nonprofit Women's Global Can-cer Alliance. His commitment is not only to screening and treatment of precancerous lesions, but to establishing a cancer registry to help direct resources, including a program to vaccinate against the cause of cervical cancer, the human papilloma virus. On his way to Minnesota to visit his father, he stopped in Iowa City where we had dinner and reminisced about Haiti. He displayed the rectitude and drive I recalled from long hours on his oncology service during residency, but he seemed to have mellowed, a trait I had not previously attributed to him.

The spectrum and diversity of struggling and suffering populations across the globe is vast. Another population of vulnerable persons is the premature infant. I have continued to follow and support the advancements which have allowed premature infants to survive. Ed Bell and his team of neonatologists at Iowa have documented this trend to offer full resuscitation and ongoing care for newborns of ever younger gestational ages at birth, some medical centers as early as 22 weeks, 18 weeks prior to a full- term pregnancy.[101] In 2000 Dr. Bell established the Tiniest Babies Registry. Though there has been increasing survivability without neurodevelopmental delay (cerebral palsy and many other disabilities), the chance for an infant to die if born between 22 and 24 weeks, or to survive with long-term adverse consequences remains high.[102] The parental decision to fully resuscitate their infants at these lower gestational ages is wrenching and must be based on the most reliable data provided by neonatologists and obstetricians acting as a team. The Neonatal Research Network, a multi-center group sponsored by NIH, updates the information upon which this counseling relies. Another major focus in Jeff Murray's laboratory has been tracking down genetic markers which may predispose a pregnancy to an early delivery.[103]

Achievements in the clinical setting, such as intact survival of 22-week infants, rely on basic science research. It has been gratifying to continue to follow the knowledge stream emanating from basic science labs. The creativity and output have been stunning. I have been particularly interested in the techniques and knowledge directed toward the development of more sophisticated mouse models, yielding greater insight into organismal development and the mechanisms by which normal embryonic and fetal development can be disrupted. These models also provide an understanding of the molecular steps which result in disease, increasing the chance for therapeutic intervention. The breadth and depth of these insights have broad applicability to our species.

Two developments which deserve mention in this context have had a profound influence on the quantity and quality of research in mice, but are impacting, and changing, many areas of biological research. One of these techniques takes advantage of the response that bacteria have developed over billions of years of evolution to combat viruses and other invading organisms. This defense is analogous to the immune reaction humans muster in response to infectious agents. To simplify, a bacterial species which carries this protective genetic material can clip off a portion of the DNA of the invading virus and insert it into its own genome in "designated" spaces. If the bacterium survives this infection, it becomes immunized against a future infection with this viral type. In a subsequent infection, the bacterium produces an RNA with homology (same sequence) to the piece of viral DNA it has stored. This RNA serves as a guide to direct a protein such as Cas9 to the same sequence in the invading virus. This protein is a nuclease which cuts the viral DNA in this spot, thus disabling the virus. Further discoveries have allowed refinements to this basic technology, usually termed CRISPR/Cas.[104] This advance was hailed as *Science* journal's Breakthrough of the Year in 2015. This technology could be likened to the significance of the development of the polymerase chain reaction (PCR) in 1985 which allows the amplification of a piece or section of DNA. PCR also borrows from the bacterial world, utilizing a bacterial protein, a DNA polymerase, which catalyzes a key step in the amplification program. The capacity to increase the quantity of fragments of dormant DNA has led to the ability, for instance, to sequence the genome of long departed hominids such as Neanderthals.

CRISPR/Cas technology, cheap and relatively easy to use, allows precise editing of genes and hence gene function, with applicability across the vast spectrum of biology. Gene knockouts in mice provide but one example. At the time of my sabbatical in 1990, KOs required making the desired genetic change in embryonic stem cells by homologous recombination, followed by methods to introduce these cells into mice and subsequent breeding trials until the desired mutation is produced. This could take a year (if fortunate) or more. Using the CRISPR/Cas approach, mice with a planned genetic modification can be produced in a fraction of this time by injection of a properly designed guide RNA and Cas9 protein into an egg or recently fertilized embryo. As a result, instructive murine models are proliferating at an accelerating pace.

Two women, Emmanuella Charpentier and Jennifer Doudna, won 2020 Nobel Prizes for their CRISPR work in bacteria. The ability to produce precise genetic modifications will extend its reach from medical research into the arenas of pest control, crops, and livestock, and even the climate.[105] An encouraging example of the use of CRISPR/Cas to ameliorate the symptoms of a debilitating genetic disease, sickle cell anemia, has been reported.[106] The desired change is initially made in blood stem cells in the laboratory prior to infusion into affected patients. The investment in intellectual capital and sheer labor that marks the progression from Oliver's 1985 demonstration that the human sickle cell locus could be targeted by homologous recombination in a pre-planned way, to the current "correction" of sickle cell disease by CRISPR/Cas technology, also relying upon the recognition of homologous sequences by an RNA introduced into the cell, has been heartening to witness.

Though the impact of CRISPR will be vast, ethical minefields are rife, the most concerning of which is the ability to change the genetic structure of embryos. Despite repeated calls from scientific organizations to abstain from crossing this boundary, He Jiankui edited the genomes of twin girls at the embryo stage of development in 2018, with the intent of rendering them resistant to HIV. This undertaking has been universally condemned. This thorny issue will likely confront us again.

A second development with a major impact on the biomedical sciences, particularly neural circuitry in the murine brain, is optogenetics, a technology which utilizes proteins called opsins, light sensitive channels which reside in cell membranes. Opsins in specialized retinal cells in the back of the eye, for instance, function as light sensors. It was shown in 2005 that these proteins can be incorporated into the cell membranes of neurons in rat brain slices. When exposed to light of a certain wavelength (depending upon the opsin), this causes the opsin channels to open and trigger "firing,"an electrical signal traveling along the length of the neuron.[107] As the field has progressed, the ability to shut neurons "off" has also been demonstrated.[108] More recently, the ability to target opsins to a selected group of neurons by viral injection into specific regions of the brains of mice and rats has allowed a plethora of studies of the neural circuits underlying behavior in these species. Again, a light source activates these channels. These electrical signals are propagated as other, linked neurons fire. These techniques have made it possible to trace neural circuits in mice which mediate behaviors such as anxiety and fear,[109] behaviors we would like to know much more about in humans. The ability to accurately edit the genome and to study neural pathways in intact animals have been powerful advances in the quest to understand normal physiological functions and the disease mechanisms by which these fail.

At this juncture it is appropriate to acknowledge a facility, the Jackson Laboratory in Bar Harbor, Maine, which has long been a national leader—and national treasure—in the field of murine genetics and service to the genetics community.[110] This independent, nonprofit has survived two fires, the first in 1947 which destroyed the facility, and one in 1987 which wiped out the mouse colony, the repository of valuable models which the laboratory distributes to investigators world-wide. Fortunately, many thousands of the facility's genetically defined strains of mice were recoverable. The laboratory is also host to a course titled Human and Mammalian Genetics and Genomics: The McKusick Short Course, begun in 1959 by Victor McKusick of Johns Hopkins University and taught by leaders in the various subdisciplines of genetics. It is almost an expected rite of passage that any card-carrying geneticist will have attended this course at least once.

Shortly after the start of the New Year in 2017 we learned of the death of Oliver Smithies at age 91. This news from Nobuyo, Oliver's wife, stated that they were walking on the beach when he collapsed and was taken to the hospital where he never regained consciousness. As Nobuyo related in her memo, he had worked through the holidays, as was his custom, and was "as spirited as usual" prior to the final event. "He was a happy man, with a lot of love for his laboratory…." A memorial service was held several months later. Field Morey, an inductee into the Wisconsin Aviation Hall of Fame, described Oliver's meticulous preparations for the record-setting flight they embarked upon. Other tributes stressed his love of science, his independent thinking, his giving qualities as a mentor, and his inclusiveness, shunning the often ego-driven and competitive nature of science. A speaker noted that one of his early signature achievements was development of starch gel electrophoresis, a method to separate proteins and DNA fragments of varying size. Until the end he designed and performed his own experiments. He was an inveterate tinkerer, inventor, and restorer. As mentioned earlier, the polymerase chain reaction (PCR) was one of those discoveries which propelled science forward. It was such an important advancement that Oliver crafted his own PCR device before their commercial availability.

Beverly Koller, Oliver's Postdoctoral student whose laborious efforts produced the first murine model of cystic fibrosis, wrote a moving essay/ obituary in a leading journal wherein she vividly captured the nature of this man.[111] She related a conversation with a colleague who told her he had attended a scientific meeting where Oliver described the first instance of homologous recombination between the mammalian genome and a piece of DNA introduced into these cells, the basis of knock-out technology before the advent of more efficient and precise gene editing technologies, notably CRISPR/Cas. The colleague told her the audience cheered as they applauded, most unusual for a normally staid group of scientists. Applause is expected; cheering is exceptional. Bev describes the piles of refurbished equipment. In the article she further relates a common vision "about how Oliver, spanner and screwdriver in hand, was known to chase down service personnel who were in the process of removing ancient equipment from the lab, hoping to salvage components for future projects." The lab reflected his character; "frugal, antiquated, and leading edge." When he died, he had been looking forward to starting a new project. In his last paper, published the year he died, he explored how the kidney prevents excretion of proteins in the blood, invoking ideas he and his mentors explored in the 1950s.[112]

In March 2021, George Bass died at age 88. Just as Oliver's former student, Bev Koller, provided a compelling account of Oliver the person and scientist, a similar obituary was published by two former students of George's, Deborah Carlson (now president of INA) and Cemal Pulak.[113] Though his death was acknowledged by pieces in the *New York Times*, *National Geographic*, and others, it was this account of his life and scholarship which resonated with me. He was a true pioneer who, with a small band of divers and archeologists, proved in the summer of 1960 that land-based standards for archeology could be applied to shipwrecks. This pioneering vision has led to the establishment of a new field of learning. He will be known by his colleagues for his innovation in devising tools and techniques, for the establishment of quality academic programs and public outreach, and for his international efforts, best exemplified by the INA Research Center in Bodrum staffed by a team of 20 Turks. He also, as his former students and colleagues attest, "always advocated for safety, simplicity, and frugality, in that order." He was also sharing, exemplified when he turned over leadership of the Uluburun shipwreck excavation, which was "the discovery of a lifetime," to his PhD student Cemal Pulak. I am grateful I knew George. He expanded my notion of learning.

In a similar manner, the repeated reference in this chapter to the sabbatical year in Chapel Hill is proportionate to its influence on my life. Having gained a deeper appreciation for basic science and the powerful molecular biology tools reflecting a growing knowledge of genetics, this led to an effort to explore and contemplate disparate fields of scientific inquiry. Science has since become even more a grounding mechanism in my life. Particularly edifying has been the attempt to understand the pervasiveness of evolution as a unifying theme for life on earth, starting with E. O. Wilson's compilation of Charles Darwin's four major treatises.[114] Darwin's sublime prose and impeccable logic in building the case for this grand theory grace the pages of these books. This overarching theme, and many other themes I have tried to convey in this personal narrative, have inspired an attempt to place this autobiographical material into a wider scientific context. Major portions of the following chapters represent "hard core" science. I have endeavored to make it accessible to laypersons with a modest background in science without, I trust, compromising the fields I will endeavor to convey.

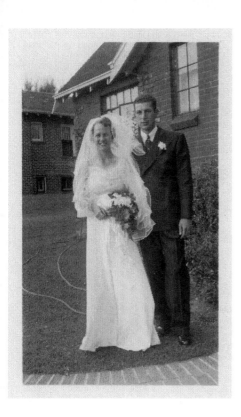

Mother and Father on their wedding day outside her father's home. This attractive picture is marred only by the hose snaking through the background.

Don Robinson supporting the author at summer camp.

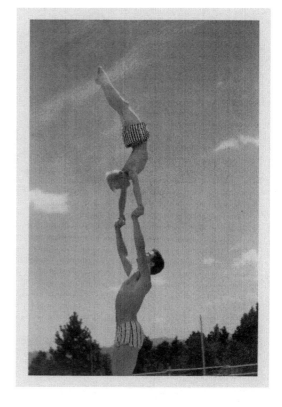

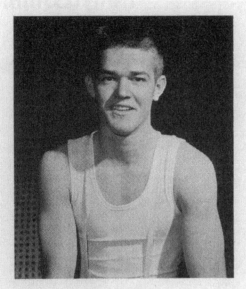

Chuck Jackson
gymnastics

Charles Jackson, the author's fraterrnity pledge father (top), and the author. Photos from fraternity files of student athletes.

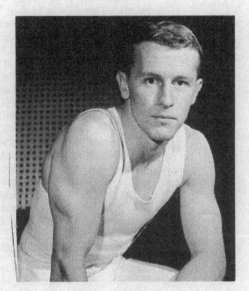

Roger Williamson
gymnastics

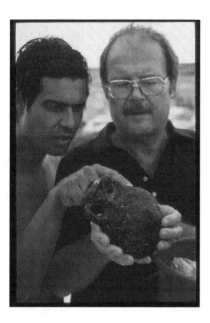

George Bass (right) and Cemal Pulak
examine a Canaanite flask excavated from the
Uluburun shipwreck. Used with permission
from the Institute of Nautical Archeology.

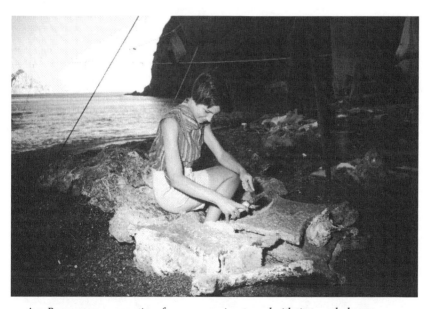

Ann Bass removes concretions from a copper ingot, used with tin to make bronze.
Ingot retrieved from the Cape Gelidonya shipwreck. Used with permission from the
Institute of Nautical Archeology.

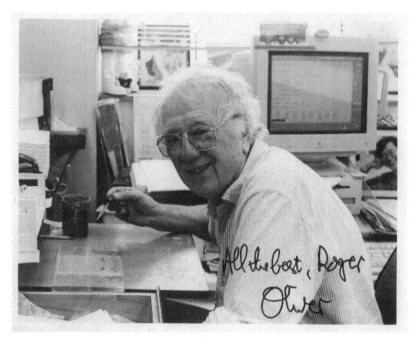

Oliver Smithies performing research at the bench.

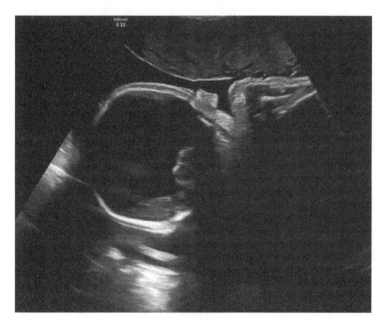

Fetus with hydranencephaly (see chapter 4). Fluid, the black area within the skull, has displaced a large portion of normal brain tissue, including the cerebral cortex. (Retrieved by the author from the Ob/Gyn ultrasound files at the University of Iowa Carver College of Medicine.)

CHAPTER TWO

Microbes
Their Complexity and Continuity

I HAVE WRITTEN A PERSONAL NARRATIVE for many reasons, but none eclipses the desire to springboard from the details of a life to fascinating realms of science, realms which may also underpin a fruitful approach to consciousness. Related to this search is the classical nature/nuture (or gene/ environment; innate/learned) dualisms which have long occupied scholars. There exists a porous divide between these dichotomies, the interchange between the astonishing abilities and propensities we are born with, inter- acting over a lifetime with the multitude of external influences we encounter.

One instance in high school was revelatory of this linkage. An inspiring biology teacher on a field trip showed her class the wriggling, darting micro- bial life within just a drop of pond water captured beneath a cover slip on a glass slide. The intense curiosity these single-celled organisms evoked has remained. Nature equipped me to appreciate the wonder of these life forms; nurture has provided the opportunity to learn about the deep biology of microbes. Though I would have been unable to define primordial at that time, microbes such as these constituted life on this planet for over 1.5 billion years before events noted below led to greater cellular complexity, the rise of multicellularity, and the subsequent exuberant diversity of organisms, living and extinct.

My purpose in this chapter is to survey the biological complexity of microorganisms, revealing some of the means and mechanisms by which these cells have evolved to establish the fundamentals upon which all of life has developed. The story encompasses basic energy generation from sophisticated nanomachines, to evolving sensory systems, to the rudiments of "cognition." These cellular building blocks have led to the establishment of a trait scholars yearn to understand, consciousness. In addition to disparate roles as foundational elements in the economy of life, microorganisms have established cycles in concert with other non-living elements which have made life on this planet possible. We are also beginning to appreciate the rich interchange between humans and their microbes consequent to colonization of our bodies, and the multiple ways this co-habitation has influenced the deep biology of our species.

⋮⋮⋮

DETAILS CONCERNING the origin of life on the planet are unknown. I have found it, nonetheless, to be a rich intellectual exercise to expose myself to the facts that are acknowledged, and to the speculations and theories which populate the gaps in our knowledge. The environment of earliest earth was harsh; a bombardment of impactors, mostly asteroids, volcanic activity, and other factors, produced searing heat. Life became possible, some would contend inevitable, when the planet cooled, crust formed, a thin layer of water appeared, and the atmosphere became more hospitable. At some point the conditions favored the transition from molecules to the first cells.

Single-celled microorganisms appear remarkably early following earth's formation from swirling gas and dust approximately 4.5 billion years ago. Though the specifics of life's origination may elude us,[1] biosignatures of living organisms and fossil evidence indicate the first microorganisms arose between 3.4–3.8 billion years ago, and possibly earlier. The geology and environmental conditions encountered by these microbes have been illuminated.[2,3] The subsequent history of these free-living cells has been a riveting story, worthy of the ongoing engagement of a once wide-eyed high schooler.

The most studied bacterium, *Escherischia coli*, has been the focus of research by many investigators, some of whom have won Nobel Prizes, including Jacob and Monod. As mentioned in the narrative preceding this portion of the book, these two scientists utilized *E. coli* to illuminate key aspects of gene regulation. The fine science writer, Carl Zimmer, has written a book on the striking capabilities of this bacterium,[4] none more so than its motoric and sensory systems for finding food. Five types of sensors are found within the forward membrane of this microorganism, each designed to detect certain molecules. When these sensors detect a food source, this signals flagella, whip-like projections from the rearward membrane. Proteins within the membrane form a complex which anchors the flagella and functions like a rotary motor. It most often turns counterclockwise, with the flagella wound into a spiral, but can instantly reverse directions by spinning clockwise, unwinding the flagella to pursue a food source or escape a predator or noxious agent. Thus, it "tumbles" from one direction to another. When the "scent" is at its peak, the bacterium will slow and feed.

Zimmer describes this behavior and many other features which have made *E. coli* the favored microbe of investigators. Though most strains of *E. coli* are harmless, a few can wreak havoc in humans. For example, so-called enteropathogenic *E. coli* can cause sometimes severe gastrointestinal (GI) disease. This strain reveals a method of obtaining nutrients while resident within the human GI tract, having evolved a device closely related to the flagellum called an injectisome. This needle-like structure can be inserted into a host cell lining the intestinal wall to extract nutrients, mostly amino acids, allowing this microbe a competitive advantage over rival microbes.[5]

Cilia and flagella are similar and show striking conservation of structure and function from protozoa to humans. Vertebrate cells have coopted and expanded upon the sensory functions of flagella. Almost every vertebrate cell projects this sensory structure, the so-called primary cilium, into the extracellular milieu to serve a variety of functions.[6] The role of cilia in sight, smell, and mechanosensation has long been known. However, the primary cilium performs other roles, including the transmission of changes in the extracellular environment to the cell interior; these signals trigger responses in many pathways, serving to integrate extracellular information and cell-cell communication. Defects in cilia cause a diverse group of serious diseases in humans.

⸙⸙⸙

HUMANS HAVE evolved from microorganisms. Throughout this process small, heritable genetic variation or change, produced randomly and passed from parent to offspring, was "scrutinized" by the process of Darwinian natural selection. The genetic change which better adapted an organism to its surroundings, allowing it to leave more progeny, passed through this selective sieve more readily. The journey from microbe to human has been rife with struggle—but also cooperativity—as transitions and thresholds were negotiated.

The earliest stages of this history have been characterized by a more fluid and communal, less complex ecological structure whereby genes were readily passed from one organism to another. This was a time of rampant horizontal gene transfer, a promiscuous sharing of genetic material. As evolution proceeded, cells became more organized and structured. Microorganisms with more defined and stable characteristics, including the ability to stifle horizontal gene transfer, gradually shifted from this mode of gene reception toward vertical transmission from parent to progeny. One of the central figures who has elucidated the large-scale organization of microbes, Carl Woese, described this transition as the "Darwinian Threshold," the time at which Darwinian natural selection became the dominant theme of evolution.[7] Horizontal gene transfer still occurs, however. One manifestation is the often devastating development of antibiotic resistance in previously susceptible microbes.

The most consequential event in this long sweep occurred approximately two billion years ago. This event was, however, not a result of small, heritable changes. Rather, one microorganism engulfed or merged with another microorganism and against what were surely prohibitive odds, the engulfed microbe became a permanent resident, eventually becoming an organelle called the mitochondrion, the structure which produces the energy to power cellular functions. This singular, fortuitous event propelled the development of multicellularity and complexity.[8,9]

This merger falls under the rubric of symbiosis, an interaction between two different organisms living in close physical association, typically to the advantage of both. These associations are common, though the vast majority do not involve the capturing and internalization of one organism by another, a process known as endosymbiosis. Lynn Margulis championed the significance of symbiosis.[10] Though some of her speculations on this subject were not correct, she was an early and steadfast defender of symbiosis as a major driver of evolution. She did not waver in the face of staunch criticism from colleagues.

Which microorganism engulfed the other, and what is the identity of the microbe which became the mitochondrion? This ongoing story is at the core of all subsequent evolutionary history. The scientist whose work defined this saga is Carl Woese, previously mentioned. He was a complicated figure whose lonely and dogged persistence over many years has provided a broad classification of the vast diversity of microorganisms based on phylogenetics, the study of evolutionary relationships developed from selected genetic sequences.

Prior to a discussion of his work, it may be helpful to review two points. First, in common biological parlance, microorganisms have been called prokaryotes, meaning cells without a membrane-enclosed nucleus which houses the chromosomes, as contrasted with eukaryotes, organisms whose cells have nuclei. The second area of review will be a woefully short primer on molecular genetics as it relates to the work of Woese. His signature research, noted below, was possible because all living cells utilize the genetic code to produce proteins, the DNA-templated strings of amino acids which carry out the functions of a cell. Protein production relies upon classes of RNA intermediates. RNA is an ancient molecule; many scholars believe life began in an "RNA world."[12, 13] Messenger or mRNA "reads" the DNA sequence (transcription), then ferries this message to the ribosomal RNA, or rRNA, where the message is translated, amino acid by amino acid, into a chain. The amino acids are delivered to rRNA by transfer RNA, or tRNA. When completed, the fully formed protein is released and transported to its site of function. Transcription and translation are the key steps when the machinery of a cell proceeds from DNA to RNA to protein.

rRNA can be readily obtained from cells in large quantities. This molecule, interacting with many proteins and tasked with translation, is so universal and essential it has been transmitted to subsequent generations of cells with little change owing to the fact that few mutations have survived selection pressures. Thus, rRNA can serve to mark lineages, an example of the utility of phylogenetics. Woese selected a particular subunit of rRNA, the 16S subunit, to assess evolutionary relationships of species of bacteria. These molecules were cut by enzymes, and the resulting smaller pieces were separated in an electrical field based on their composition. The pieces had been labeled by a radioactive tag which allowed them to be visualized on X-ray film, producing dark spots on the developed radiograph. Over the years Woese had become familiar with the patterns, or "fingerprints," of over 100 bacterial species.

Well into his investigations in the 1970s at the University of Illinois at Urbana, a colleague at the same institution offered Woese an unusual organism to study, a member of a group called "methanogens." Methanogens produce methane as a byproduct of hydrogen and carbon dioxide metabolism in anaerobic (lacking oxygen) environments. Microorganisms living in these environments are difficult to grow in the lab and, hence, had been little studied. Woese subjected the organism to his fingerprinting technique. He knew the patterns of dark spots on the X-ray films that bacteria displayed. Thus, when the pattern emerged for this methanogen, he could readily discern that certain spots in the radiograph indicative of bacteria were missing, and others not seen in bacteria were present. This allowed Woese to declare he had discovered a heretofore unknown Domain he termed Archaebacteria.[11] At that time, he interpreted archaea to be a third Domain; the other two were Bacteria and Eukaryota. This immensely consequential finding was doubted and roundly dismissed for about a decade until other data corroborated his findings. Woese, naturally reticent, became withdrawn and embittered, though he continued to combatively defend his findings.

This story and its significance have become more involved (and fascinating). Though bacteria and archaea are similar in many ways, including their appearance under a microscope, they differ in their habitats and, as alluded, their genetic structure. Whereas bacteria are ubiquitous, archaea are often found in extreme environments; hence their frequent designation as "extremophiles." Some are hyperthermophilic, preferring the extremely high temperatures of undersea hydrothermal vents or hot springs. Some have adapted to the extremes of pH (from acid to alkaline) found on earth, while others are "halophiles," living in conditions of high salt concentration, and still others are "barophiles," existing on and under the sea floor, including the deepest ocean reaches, at crushing pressures. Other archaea may live a more prosaic existence in the human gut where they join a plethora of bacterial species, fungi, and viruses.

A discussion of microorganisms again invites the question: how did life originate and under what conditions? Theories abound. Creative possibilities include importation of life beyond our planet, but that only pushes the origin back in time. Arguments for a beginning in undersea hydrothermal vents make this a top contender. Facts have been marshalled which plausibly support an origin at these vents and suggest experiments that could get us closer to acceptance or refutation of this theory.[14, 15]

In 2015, archaea were collected near hydrothermal vents in the deep ocean near Greenland, vents known as Loki's Castle, named for the troublemaker Norse god Loki. Though these microbes could not be cultured at this time, microbial DNA recovered from the seafloor sediment was sequenced. Using metagenomic analyses to piece together the sequenced fragments, a newly discovered archael species was documented with a set of core genes phylogenetically related to corresponding genes in eukaryotes.[16] Genomic information collected from other archael species has confirmed that suites of genes within this domain are closely related to a core set of genes in eukaryotes. Based upon these findings, investigators in the field have been seriously considering that there are not three domains, but rather two, and that eukaryotes like fungi, plants, and humans arose within a lineage of the archael domain.[17]

A major breakthrough has been the recovery of archael species from seafloor mud by a Japanese submersible in waters near Japan. After a 12-year effort, attempting to simulate the conditions in which it lived, an archael species has been cultured in the laboratory.[18] This will allow more sophisticated studies, such as investigations into the metabolism of these organisms. The Japanese team again documented that this archael species expressed what have been termed "eukaryote signature genes." As other species of archaea are cultured and studied in the lab, it is likely we will accumulate sufficient evidence to definitively know if we are descended from archaea.

As mentioned, about two billion years ago a microbe engulfed a fellow microbe. Genomic studies identify this latter microbe as a bacterium, an alphaproterobacteria. Current research also indicates that the engulfing host cell was an archeon. This was, as previously stated, a singular event. Over time the endosymbiont (now mitochondrion) either lost or transferred most of its genes to the host genome. The transferred genes manufactured proteins which could then be transported back to the mitochondria to help build and maintain the intricate complex of molecular structures which produce energy.

Doubtless there was inherent conflict following this endosymbiosis. However, it should also be noted that environmental conditions may have favored accommodation or cooperativity between host and endosymbi-ont. Around the time of this symbiosis, the oxygen levels on earth were rising, largely due to the production of oxygen by cyanobacteria. To survive rising oxygen levels, anaerobic archaea would have to adjust. This adjustment may have been facilitated by the presence of oxygen-utilizing mitochondria. Analogous to energy generation by mitochondria, cyanobacteria became the photosynthesizing organelle of plants, the chloroplast, following endosymbiosis.

⁂

MOST OF US are keenly interested in origin stories. David Quammen has written an accessible account of the remarkable history of early life on earth and one man's perseverance in documenting the existence of archaea.[19] He relates in lucid detail the early history of extensive gene sharing, horizontal gene transfer, and the subsequent efforts fueling the debate about the progenitor cell from which humans may have evolved. Quammen presents a more nuanced portrait of Woese, a person noted for his prickly personality. In another corrective on the life of Woese, former colleagues noted that co-workers and friends found him "brilliant, witty, brutally honest, generous, and humble."[20]

Bacteria and archaea have remained relatively unchanged since horizontal gene transfer ceased to be the dominant feature of the genomic landscape. However, during this early period of DNA swapping, these cells acquired genes for the assembly of remarkable nanomachines that persist in the cells of all living organisms. This collective gene pool included those coding for the construction of ribosomes, utilized by Carl Woese to delineate bacteria and archaea. Also included in this genetic mélange were instructions to build other sophisticated nanomachines that plants acquired through the merger of the ancestor of plants with a cyanobacterium, precursor of the chloroplast, and that other organisms acquired with the merger that resulted in the mitochondrion. Plants manufacture carbohydrates from carbon dioxide and water, utilizing the energy from sunlight captured by chlorophyll. Oxygen, critically important for all of life not living in anaerobic habitats, is released as a byproduct of photosynthesis. As mentioned, oxygen is utilized by mitochondria in the process of energy generation.

Mitochondria and other nanomachines operating within the vast diversity of microorganisms have enabled the favorable environmental conditions on earth that have supported life. These microbes have done so while inhabiting terrestrial and aquatic niches worldwide, some under extreme circumstances.[21] Paul Falkowski has written extensively on biogeochemical cycles, the multiple loops of interaction along the abiotic and biotic spectrums of the production and consumption of energy and materials.[22, 23]

The materials that are supplied to these interaction loops are derived from the atmosphere, the mantle and crust, ocean sediments, and tectonic plate activity. These materials reciprocally interact with the array of microbial bioenergetic and metabolic processes. Many of the intricacies of these interconnected pathways are yet to be worked out, but the perpetuation of life on this planet is unquestionably reliant upon microorganisms, the bedrock of this grand enterprise.

At the scale of atoms, these nanomachines drive the reactions upon which these biogeochemical processes depend. The redox reaction is the underpinning of these processes, and the movement of electrons is the basis of the redox reaction. Redox couples the reduction or loss of electrons with the gain of electrons or oxidation; the electron donor becomes oxidized, and the electron acceptor becomes reduced. Redox reactions undergird the biogeochemical cycles described in broad outline in the previous paragraph. The other key component of bioenergetics, the movement of energy throughout a cell, is a consequence of the flux of protons across a bioenergetic membrane.

Nick Lane and others have deeply considered how mitochondria function, leading, in the consideration of many, to the development of the nucleus, sex, two sexes, aging, and apoptosis, a process/phenomenon of cell death critical for embryological development and health.[9,15] The nanomachines within the hundreds to thousands of mitochondria per cell perform the feat of energy generation by utilizing the two charged particles of an atom, the negatively charged electron and positively charged proton.

Mitochondria are surrounded by an inner and outer membrane. Residing within the inner membrane is the bacterially acquired machinery to produce adenosine triphosphate (ATP), storing energy for cellular functions in high-energy phosphate bonds. This machinery consists of a series or chain of multi-protein reaction or redox centers. Protons and electrons are first stripped from the remains of the food we consume. The electrons are passed or transferred down this chain within the inner membrane. Waiting at the end of this chain is oxygen with a strong avidity for electrons, propelled through these complexes by this attractive force. The manner by which these electrons flow has, according to Lane, characteristics of particle movement in the quantum world. "Electrons hop from centre to centre. In fact, the regular spacing of these centres suggests that electrons 'tunnel' by some form of quantum magic, appearing and disappearing fleetingly, according to the rules of quantum probability."[15] (p. 69)

The current of electrons moving toward oxygen powers the extrusion of protons from the innermost mitochondrial compartment (matrix) to the space between the inner and outer membranes. This produces an electrical potential across the membrane. When oxygen molecules combine with electrons after final electron transfer, protons move back across the membrane, following the electrochemical gradient, and enter a protein complex called ATP synthase. This ancient assemblage, conserved in all organisms, functions like a rotary motor. The flux of protons back through ATP synthase turns this motor to produce ATP.

This movement of protons to ATP synthase turns this motor much like water cascading onto a water wheel turns its paddles to generate a power source. Proton-motive force arose very early and is widespread in nature. The motors which propel the flagella of *E. coli*, for instance, are driven by proton-motive force. The individual who conceived this counterintuitive, unexpected notion, and proved it through experimentation in a laboratory he built in his home, was Peter Mitchell.[24] His findings were met with initial skepticism and considerable opposition. The centrality of proton-motive force within a cell was ultimately accepted, and he won the Nobel Prize in 1978.

Much in this realm of energy generation remains unexplained. Lane leaves us with questions that will compel experimentation for a considerable time. "We now know that these ideas are true; but are we any closer to knowing why they are true? The question boils down to two parts: why do all cells use redox chemistry as a source of free energy? And why do all cells conserve this energy in the form of proton gradients over membranes? At a more fundamental level, why electrons and why protons?"[15] (p. 77) Nature uses the materials at hand; for these key life processes the most fundamental of materials, the particles of an atom, have been procured.

So much has been enabled in single-celled microorganisms by electrons and protons. Relatively recent observations have revealed another novel example of redox behavior. Bacteria, living on the sea floor in shallow waters with access to oxygen, can form a mutually beneficial consortium with microbes living in anoxic conditions only millimeters to a few centimeters beneath the sea floor. The relationship involves transfer of electrons through filamentous nanowires projecting from the surfaces of one species of the consortium to the other, enabling vital metabolic processes in both species.[25] This is yet another example of the redox mechanisms which have evolved within the biogeochemical capabilities of microbes. This may be the earliest trace of the development of communication within organisms possessing nervous systems.

While intercellular communication via electrons appears uncommon in microorganisms, a unique form of chemical communication called quorum sensing (QS) is prevalent within the microbial world.[26] Bacteria avidly attach to moist surfaces supplied with nutrients. These bacteria have an elaborate system of information sharing via chemical signals. These signals are received by receptors on cell membranes. As the microbes multiply, a biofilm develops. Stream rocks, teeth, pipes, and wounds are among favored surfaces for biofilm formation. As biofilms establish a communication network, the structures take on aspects of multicellularity. At some point in the growth of a biofilm a "quorum" is reached. What triggers this awareness is not known. However, at this point the signals switch functions and begin to activate batteries of genes to serve multiple other purposes; for instance, to control growth of the biofilm, form spores, produce toxins against host cells or other virulence factors against rival microorganisms, or to initiate bioluminescence or light emission.

Bioluminescence is a particularly interesting capability. Some species of luminous bacteria form symbiotic relationships with fish and squid. The light from bacteria aids the host in finding food and mates, and evading predators. The host provides the bacteria a suitable growing environment. Bioluminescence in the Hawaiian bobtail squid is a vivid demonstration of QS in the service of defense. The bacteria, *Vibrio fischeri*, living in the squid's specialized light organ, uniquely protect the squid from predators when it feeds at night near the surface. These bacteria multiply and, when a certain population threshold density is reached, they begin to glow,[27] tuning the bioluminescence to that of the moon's radiance and starlight to shield the squid from predators below. As stated, the genes controlling bioluminescence are not activated until a quorum is achieved, thus conserving energy. At dawn the squid burrows into a sandy bottom and discharges the bacteria. As night approaches they again gather *Vibrio fischeri* bacteria.

Within growing biofilms, cooperative behavior often manifests, leading to metabolic co-dependence. As *Bacillus subtilis* biofilms grow, the interior of this expanded colony becomes starved for nutrients. To preserve colony fitness, the signals from the interior to peripheral cells and back periodically halt growth of the biofilm, allowing interior cells access to nutrients.[28] These coordinated oscillations lead to a more resilient colony. Most microorganisms exist within social contexts which feature a mix of cooperation, as noted in the example of *B. subtilis*, and competition.[29]

Biofilms impacting medicine are intensively studied to achieve effective treatments. Prevalent among the extant examples is the propensity of the pathogen *Pseudomonas aruginosa* to form biofilms on the lung surfaces of individuals with cystic fibrosis. Affected individuals have difficulty clearing secretions from their airways, making them vulnerable to infection. In the long history of battles waged against microorganisms, deterrence advances by the host beget appropriate/effective defense strategies by the intruder; this ratcheted process is relentless. *Pseudomonas* infection exemplifies the way host cells can "spy" upon the developmental stage and virulence of its biofilm.[30] Host cells have developed receptors on their surfaces to bind to and thus monitor the activity of the biofilm's QS molecules. This provides the host knowledge which will modulate or tune its immune response to the infection. This type of surveillance is not the exception but the rule. An understanding of the defense mechanisms the host employs may assist the development of therapeutics.

In addition to bacterial cooperation exemplified by QS, bacteria can also instruct in another realm that social scientists investigate in human interactions. Cheating is a potent counter to cooperation. Bacterial "cheaters" do not produce QS signals, thus conserving energy. However, they do take advantage of the nutritional and defense properties conferred by QS. When cheaters were mixed with a wild-type strain of *P. aeruginosa*, the cheaters exploited the advantages to the detriment of the colony.[31] Microbes have developed a wide range of strategies to deter cheaters.[32]

Considering so many behaviors displayed by microorganisms, fashioned from an internal genetic program interacting with their environment, these discussions of genetic and environmental contributions are not unlike those evoked by the field of Sociobiology, founded by E. O. Wilson.[33] The parallels with animal behavior are sufficiently compelling for some to apply the label "Sociomicrobiology"[34] to the wiles and machinations of microbes.

Most of the QS chemical signals are diffusible and are released without "packaging." *Pseudomonas aeruginosa* and other bacteria can, however, use a different strategy for delivering poorly soluble signaling molecules. These, including antibiotics against competing bacteria and toxins against host cells to aid the *P. aeruginosa* infection, can be packaged into membranous vesicles and released.[35] By this means, these "bacterial speech bubbles" can signal more distant cells to carry out the packaged instructions.

These sophisticated communication systems and other adaptations that bacteria utilize invites the question: can any behaviors of bacteria be considered "cognitive?" Can we infer that bacteria are capable of memory, learning, and anticipation? Several studies suggest affirmative evidence (reviewed[36]). The bacterium *E. coli* confronts diverse environmental conditions during its life cycle, from soil and sediment to water and GI tracts. The transition to the mammalian GI tract involves a rise in temperature in the oral cavity, followed directly by a drop in oxygen concentration in the anaerobic GI tract. Under these simulated laboratory circumstances, activation of a genetic program—the heat shock response when oral cavity temperature is simulated—is tightly coupled to repression of genes for aerobic respiration, rapidly reprogramming to an anaerobic mode as *E. coli* enters the gut. When these circumstances are reversed, simulating excretion from the GI tract, these genetic programs are rapidly reversed.[37] This coupling suggests a tight link has been established between signal transduction pathways, enabling the microbes to anticipate environmental circumstances and rapidly respond.

The evolution of another remarkable system for integrating signals from beyond the cell boundary was initiated in the bacterial world, the development of an internal, 24-hour clock. The predictable day/night sunlight generated by the earth's rotation cue physiological changes in cyanobacteria, precursor of the plant chloroplast, to regulate functional output in this bacterium based on the time of the day.[38] This microbe accomplishes this with three proteins which cycle in a predictable manner.[39] Of all bacteria capable of some form of photosynthesis, only cyanobacteria generate oxygen.[40]

Early pioneering observers[41, 42] launched investigations into the internal clocks of many model systems, including fungi, flies, birds, and mammals, earning Jeffrey Hall, Michael Robash, and Michael Young Nobel Prizes in 2017. Research over the past several decades has revealed the molecular intricacies of circadian rhythm cycling which governs sleep, feeding, the cell cycle, metabolism, hormonal cycling, immune function, migration, and hibernation. These clocks cycle in a cell-autonomous fashion, meaning the function is intrinsic to the cell. The components driving the process are the oscillators, the proteins which act on "clock genes" to produce positive and negative elements comprising feedback loops. The positive elements of the loop rise and stimulate production of negative elements which, in turn, inhibit production of positive elements. When the negative elements undergo decay, the cycle begins again with production of the positively acting proteins.[43] From these feedback loops have emerged the oscillators which sustain this repetitive variation in cellular output. Diverse organisms have evolved diverse clocks, though within mammals, for instance, the implicated genes are highly conserved.

The anatomy of this time keeping system is also highly conserved among mammals. The paired suprachiasmatic nuclei within the hypothalamus contain neurons which receive neural signals from the retina in the back of the eye. Collectively, these neurons function as an oscillator which is entrained (synchronized) by light. Though nearly every cell in the body has genes encoding a circadian clock, only the neurons in the hypothalamus are known to be synchronized by light. The autonomous oscillators of cellular clocks throughout the body are coordinated by the "master clock" in the suprachiasmatic nuclei. This ensures that the gene networks within cells involved in metabolism and the redox or energetic status of the cell,[44] as well as other functions, including immune function,[45] cycle in a coordinated fashion that benefits the entire organism. It is not surprising that sleep disturbances, depression, and metabolic disorders are associated with altered circadian rhythms.[46] One study documented a cyclic (circadian) rise and fall in about 100 gene products in post-mortem samples from six regions of the brains of normal human subjects. There was a breakdown in this pattern in patients with major depressive disorder.[47] Much more work is required.

A study in mice showed that regulation of genes in the suprachiasmatic nuclei and an organ at the hub of metabolism, the liver, cycle circadianly, optimizing metabolic activity to the most useful time of the day.[48] Extrapolating their findings to other organs, the authors estimate that around 10 percent of the mammalian transcriptome (a read out of the genes which have been transcribed) may be under circadian control.

As is evident from the foregoing, microbes display sophisticated systems as these cells negotiate their environments. Many microbial activities are precursors of those we witness in more "evolved" organisms. Microbes, like all cells, maintain an electrical gradient across their membranes, allowing nutrients to move to the interior and waste to be eliminated. The ability to sense light, temperature, and nutrients heralded the later development of sensory systems based on electrical transmission. Neurons and nervous systems have antecedents in microorganisms that became modified as small genetic changes were selected for their utility and survival value. These hints of greater complexity led to intermediate structures, such as the neural nets of jellyfish, to the organization of neurons transmitting messages over membranous neural tracts. Electrical transmission—in the form of action potentials—proceeds down the axonal membranes of neurons to the synaptic cleft. A neurotransmitter released within this cleft facilitates the continuation of the action potential to the next neuron in the pathway. Neurotransmitters can be as simple as an amino acid. This chemical messaging harkens back to behavioral traits in microbes mediated by quorum sensing.

⋄⋄⋄

MICROBES, as has been stated, were the only living entities on the planet for over 1.5 billion years. As other organisms made their appearance, microbes were in the unfamiliar position of sharing the world. And share they did! Just as they have occupied the available worldwide niches, microbes have inhabited nearly every ecological niche provided by earth's emerging co-inhabitants. Microbes in massive numbers, many trillions, live on or within the bodies of animals, particularly the GI tract. Though there are many commonalities, the species composition is different in all individuals. In humans, over 1,000 microbial species exist in the GI tract,[49] with about 7,000 strains.[50] As they have taken up residence, microbes have been immensely impactful. They have had to adapt to and co-exist with myriad other microorganisms, including viruses, fungi, and parasites.[51] Many consider a host and their microbes a "holobiont," a dynamic ecosystem with bidirectional influences from microorganisms to host and back.

Efforts are underway to evaluate the genetic diversity of human microbes, the microbiome.[49, 52] These studies have revealed hundreds of genes absent from the human genome.[53] These metagenomic studies do not capture small genes for methodologic and computational reasons. However, when specifically searched for, a recent study defined greater than 4,000 such genes, most of unknown function, though about 30 percent of the protein families coded by these genes were predicted to be secreted, implicating them in cell-to-cell communication.[54] This chemical messaging would presumably serve numerous purposes within this collective conglomerate, analogous to quorum sensing within a biofilm. As we learn more about the overall genetic structure of the microbiome, we are also beginning to ferret out the molecular mechanisms that allow cooperation among species within the microbiome.[55]

Though the gut can be a target of infectious agents, the vast majority of the teeming GI microbial community are commensal, deriving nutrition from the host without causing harm. Many species are critically helpful in the digestion of food and development of the immune system. A metagenomic analysis of GI microbes has revealed genes which produce vitamins and complement host genes in breaking down dietary fiber and metabolizing drugs, amino acids, and other compounds.[52] Studies in mice raised in germ-free colonies have uncovered a role of microbes in energy storage and utilization.[56] When germ-free mice received gut microbes from conventionally raised mice, the body fat content of these mice increased by 60 percent.

Maternal health, including diet, influences the fetal environment and can program fetal physiology. This programming may predispose to diseases such as hypertension, cardiac disease, and diabetes later in life. This process of fetal programming, known as the Barker hypothesis,[57] has generally been applied to humans, wherein many examples could be cited. Fetal programming, for example, may be operative within the observation that, in humans, maternal obesity and diabetes increases the risk for offspring to develop autism.[58] A cardinal feature of autism is deficits in the social realm. Murine models have again been instructive in this context. Mice are social animals, and relatively straightforward observations can discern levels of murine social interaction. When pregnant female mice are fed a high-fat diet during pregnancy, their offspring similarly showed social deficits when tested three to eight weeks after weaning.[59] There were changes in the gut microbiomes of these mice compared to those born to mothers on a normal diet. There were also fewer neurons in the hypothalamus that produce oxytocin, a hormone known to facilitate social interactions in humans.[60]

In this study,[59] if the gut microbiomes of affected mice were reconstituted from normal mice, or if the mice with social deficits were housed with normal mice, thereby receiving passive transfer of a normal microbiome, the social deficits resolved, and oxytocin levels normalized. The authors isolated a microbial species, *Lactobacillus reuteriis*, which could reverse the deficits. They surmised this species released a metabolite or peptide that possibly traveled to the brain via the vagus nerve, a long bidirectional tract connecting the brainstem to multiple organs, including the GI tract.

The research group that studied the consequences of a high-fat diet fed to pregnant mice[59] has, more recently, evaluated three more murine models of autism spectrum disorder (ASD).[61] In one of these models, a gene implicated in human ASD, Shank3B, was inactivated via gene targeting, a methodology discussed in the personal narrative. These mice exhibit behaviors seen in human ASD patients, including social deficits and repetitive behaviors. The study again documented that the bacterium *L. reuteriis* reversed the social deficits. Detailed studies have begun to reveal how this bacterium impacts brain function. Their findings pointed to the social reward circuits involving oxytocin and dopamine pathways. When synapses in pathways are functional and are stimulated, they show electrical changes interpreted as plasticity. Learning and other neural functions are dependent upon plasticity, the property that allows change within the relevant circuits. In these murine models of ASD, this plasticity in the reward pathways is absent. Lastly, it was shown in this study that the efficacy of *L. reuteriis* is mediated by the vagus nerve. If the vagus nerve is severed, this bacterium is ineffective in ameliorating the social deficits.

Studies that support a gut-brain axis are multiplying. We are learning that there is a relationship between an organism's microbiome and social behavior across a wide span of organisms, including termites, flies, zebrafish, rodents, and primates.[62] In animal models wherein the behavior can be assessed, the microbiome influences communication, learning and memory, and behavioral outcomes such as anxiety and depression, often accompanied by concomitant neurophysiological correlates of these traits.[63] These studies demonstrate that the long co-evolution of animals and microbes has influenced functions of the central nervous system.

Further evidence that coevolution of mammals and their microbiomes can affect normal brain development and behavior is starkly demonstrated by mice raised in germ-free conditions. As adults, these mice show decreased anxiety and increased motor activity.[64] It seems that for anxiety to develop in mice, microbial colonization is required. If germ-free mice are provided normal gut microbes early in life, baseline levels of anxiety and motor activity are observed. In this study, there were accompanying alterations in the expression of relevant genes in areas of the brain involved in motor activity and anxiety in these germ-free mice.

Investigations in mice showing that gut microbes can affect mental state, and suggestive studies in humans involving small numbers, have led to more robust investigations to understand the relationship between microbial metabolism and psychological health. A study with large numbers, over 1,000 Dutch and over 1,000 Belgium citizens, independently showed that those with well documented depression were missing two species of bacteria, *Coprococcus* and *Dialister*, from their microbiomes.[65] The authors compiled a list of 56 neuroactive chemicals that microbes either produce or metabolize. One substance they identified with *Coprococcus* is a metabolite of dopamine, one of the brain neurotransmitters which has been implicated in depression. The authors were not able to determine if this bacterium manufactures this metabolite or produces it by breaking down dopamine.

Before turning to a discussion of immunity, several comments impacting our current understanding of the association between the microbiome and human health are warranted. The reported increases in the incidence of disorders of immunity (e.g., asthma and inflammatory bowel disease), metabolism (e.g., obesity and diabetes), and cognition (e.g., autism spectrum disorder) have been linked to the microbiome,[66] though much work remains to ferret out the mechanisms involved. This has spawned the probiotic industry, ingesting living microbes with the intent of altering the gut microbiome to achieve a favorable therapeutic effect. Unfortunately, probiotics have not been rigorously studied, though there remains the potential of targeted alterations of the assemblage of gut microbes to combat some of these disorders.

Another issue which has garnered attention is the "hygiene hypothesis," the thesis that the current emphasis on cleanliness has deprived infants of exposure to an array of environmental agents, including microbes, thus thwarting the development of protective immunity. Martin Blaser argues against this explanation for the rising incidence of the disease categories cited. His argument focuses on the overuse of antibiotics and the consequential elimination of beneficial microbes.[67] He also describes the acquisition of the microbes which begin inhabiting the bodies of newborns at birth. The composition differs depending upon route of delivery, vaginal versus Cesarean section. In the U.S., the rate of Cesarean section delivery has risen significantly. Though the microbiomes of babies born by either route tend to converge over time, the author is concerned that Cesarean section delivery will disrupt the beneficial bidirectional influences among vaginally acquired microbes and immunity, metabolism, and cognition at a critical time in development of the cellular processes underlying these systems. The consequences, he postulates, could be like those resulting from the overuse of antibiotics.[67] These studies are ongoing.

⁂

I BEGAN this chapter with mention of the biology we are born with, the innate physical and mental abilities we possess, and those we acquire as we live out our lives enmeshed within our environments. Immunity cogently exemplifies these biological pathways. The two arms of the immune system are referred to as the innate and acquired (adaptive) immune systems. Both have evolved to distinguish self from non-self. Though the immune system responds to many environmental challenges, the principal targets are microbial, distinguishing harmful species—which will elicit a reaction to neutralize or destroy—from the vast majority of benign (or even helpful) microorganisms.

Innate immunity is ancient. It has evolved by natural selection over the vast history during which multicellular organisms have been associated with infectious microbes. The central elements of innate immunity are the receptors within host membranes that recognize distinct patterns of molecules produced by microbes. These receptors, called Toll or Toll-like receptors, recognize and bind elements within these molecular patterns—called pathogen-associated molecular patterns (PAMPs). Infectious and non-infectious microbes produce PAMPs, but the innate receptors have become "programmed" to initiate a protective response only when binding those of infectious agents. These patterns have not changed over eons because they are essential to a pathogen's ability to infect, and hence survive.

This lack of change provided the host immune system the opportunity to develop invariant receptor types to recognize these invariant PAMPs.

Importantly, one component of this innate immune response is activation of the other arm, adaptive immunity. This adaptive system learns to mount a response by exposure throughout life to offending antigens, proteins from many sources, not just microbes, which can cause harm. The adaptive system, present in all jawed vertebrates, features two types of lymphocytes, T and B cells. When both arms of the immune system are involved, communication flows back and forth to combat microbes. As is the case for the innate system, the key component of the adaptive immune system is the antigen receptor on the surface of T and B cells. These receptors are assembled from segments of the genome which have been encoded in the germline (eggs and sperm), but which are rearranged and recombined to produce a vast and diverse array of receptors. These are randomly produced after birth in such large numbers that virtually any antigen can be recognized by this dynamic system. When an antigen is engaged, that population of T or B cell expands considerably, referred to as clonal expansion.

B and T cells work in concert, though their functions differ. B cells produce antibodies against microbes following an infection. They also retain a memory of that encounter and will rapidly respond if reinfection occurs with the same agent. T cells undergo a process of education in the thymus (central education of T cells as opposed to peripheral education). T cells which are self-reactive—with the potential to cause autoimmunity—are eliminated. However, a small subset of self-reactive T cells can be differentiated in the thymus into a type of regulatory T cell which will not react against host tissues. These cells and those T cells with receptors directed against non-self are selected, leave the thymus, and begin to patrol the body for foreign antigens.

The immune system is an organization of cells and molecules exquisitely tuned to combat harmful microbes.[68] The innate system does not retain a memory of previous infections and, hence, reacts to an offending microbe in the same manner with each encounter. In contrast, the adaptive immune system, upon a repeat encounter, reacts rapidly with the same targeted response. In 2011 three investigators won Nobel Prizes for discovering key features of these two immune systems. Ralph Steinman revealed the cell, the dendritic cell, which detects invaders via PAMPs, producing antigens after they ingest the microbe.[69] The dendritic cells then travel to the regional lymph nodes where they present the specific antigen on their cell surface. When a T lymphocyte with the cognate (related) receptor encounters and binds the antigen, this begins a cascade of immune responses.

Two decades after the discovery of the role of dendritic cells, Jules Hoffman was investigating the reason fruit flies, without an adaptive immune system, could survive fungal infections. His group[70] and that of Bruce Beutler[71] had independently discovered the Toll gene, also known to be involved in fly development. This receptor initiates the immune response protecting the flies. The Toll or Toll-like receptor mediates the innate immune response. Some form of innate immunity probably exists in all multicellular organisms. Toll receptors exist exclusively for combating infectious microbes, whereas a variety of agents, as mentioned, trigger the adaptive response.

It may be of interest to also note that the microorganisms against which this innate and adaptive immune arsenal is arrayed have their own challenges, principally viruses. In response, bacteria and archaea have developed both innate and adaptive defense mechanisms. Both domains of microorganisms possess so-called restriction endonucleases, enzymes which will cut invading viral DNA or RNA when these enzymes recognize a specific string of bases within the viral genetic material. This is one of the innate defenses these microbes possess. Research in the 1970s revealed the potential to utilize these enzymes to recombine genomes. This precipitated a major controversy, resulting in the Recombinant DNA Conference at Asilomar in California in 1975. The emphasis was on biocontainment and biosecurity. This conference was a model for what has become more widespread public, legal, ethical, and governmental involvement with the burgeoning genetic technologies.

It has only been relatively recently determined that most archaea and many bacteria also have an adaptive immune system called CRISPR/ Cas. As noted in the personal narrative, this defensive system functions by incorporating fragments of viral DNA into CRISPR sites of a bacterial or archael genome upon first infection. If the microbe survives this attack, it uses the transcripts of these unique viral sequences to target and inactivate the cognate regions of the viral genome upon reinfection with the same virus.[72] Specific immunity had been acquired at the time of the first infection. Accordingly, the CRISPR-Cas defenses of bacteria and archaea fulfill the definition of adaptive immunity.

While microbes are battling opponents with their own sophisticated immune systems, one might reasonably ask why humans and other mammals do not just reject the lot of them? After all, the antigenic profile of microbes is significantly different from host antigens. This is a query not unlike asking why mothers do not reject their fetuses with whom they share half of their genes, guaranteeing their fetus will have "foreign" antigens. These scientific conundrums have spurred considerable research and suggestive, but not definitive, answers.

Evidence to date favors the conclusion that both the host innate and adaptive immune systems, in concert with the trillions of microorganisms, have co-evolved as a "superorganism" invested in the integrity of the mucosal gut lining. Inflammation or a breach of this lining leaves the host and its commensal microbes vulnerable. A cooperative, symbiotic network between host and microbiome has been formed that, for the most part, keeps the less than 100 microbes which are truly infectious under control.

When considering the relationships among microbes and mammalian immune systems, it should be noted that germ-free mice have an underdeveloped immune system with adverse consequences for these animals (reviewed [73]). It also appears that the expected colonization shortly after birth is the "window of opportunity" to establish a normally functioning immune system.[74] The dependence of immune system development on the microbiome is clear.

The microbiome is essential to good health. How, though, has accommodation to these interlopers been accomplished? Again, the answers are not fully known. It had earlier been thought that microbes were sequestered within the mucosal gut lining, thus preventing an inflammatory host response. The view over the last several decades is that host and microbiome interact in a manner that keeps infectious microbes at bay and supports the remainder of the microbiome. Both infectious microbes and commensals display molecular patterns (PAMPs) that can be recognized by Toll-like receptors on immune cells and receptors associated with the GI tract lining. Entire classes of microbes share the large number of molecular patterns that are recognized by a relatively small number of Toll-like receptors we are born with. This recognition and binding not only allows defense against infectious microbes, but also recognition of commensal PAMPs which protect the lining against breaches and inflammation.[75] A differential immune response to these two classes maintains a steady state physiology or homeostasis in the GI tract.

There is also significant interchange between the adaptive immune system and commensal microbes in the GI tract. Recall that T cells undergo an early sorting in the thymus. This instruction involves elimination of self-reactive T cells to prevent autoimmunity. There is also a small subset of potentially self-reactive T cells that are differentiated within the thymus into a self-tolerant regulatory T cell. One study evaluated the possibility that a population of T cells generated in the periphery may be rendered tolerant of microbes in the gut when exposed to their antigens, a means to avoid inflammatory bowel disease.[76] Indeed, microbial instruction of peripheral T cells causes a shift to regulatory T cells with receptors which allow peaceful accommodation to a variety of non-self-antigens derived from the commensal microbes.

These and similar findings have led investigators to contend that our microbiota has had a major role in the evolution of the adaptive immune system.[71] Invertebrates do not have an adaptive immune system, but also have small numbers of resident microbes. It is possible the innate immune system of invertebrates without memory is sufficient to "manage." In contrast vertebrates, particularly mammals, harbor great numbers of microbes. Therefore, an adaptive immune system with memory of past encounters may be required to derive mutual benefit and avoid harm.[77]

These systems in our bodies are so interwoven it is not surprising that attention is increasingly turning to the mutual connections which have been elaborated over an extended period, not just between the microbiota and immune systems, but among these entities and the peripheral and central nervous systems (CNS). Aspects of these interactions have been highlighted in this chapter. The CNS has an extensive immune system with many of the characteristics heretofore noted. This contrasts with older views that the CNS was immune-privileged. The recent demonstration of a CNS lymphatic system to channel immune cells and molecules expands our view of the influential role the immune system may play in the CNS.[78] The gut microbiota plays an integral role in mediating neuroimmune interactions that impact disorders such as anxiety and depression, and others.

The immune modulation extends to neurogenesis or production of new neurons, as well as the neurotransmitters synthesized in the CNS and in peripheral tissues, including synthesis of neurotransmitters by microbes. Psychological stress activates the hypothalamus-pituitary-adrenal axis to release glucocorticoids such as cortisol. This compound has major effects on immunity as well as the intestinal tract and its inhabitants. These interactions that constitute a gut-immune-CNS axis have been reviewed.[79]

Microbes and immune and nervous systems are thoroughly integrated into the economies of our bodies. Words utilized or implied in this chapter such as "instruction," "learning," "education," and "memory" have heuristic value when describing the interactions of these systems at the cellular level. It is not overreaching to suggest that our cells, over the vastness of time, have become greatly modified microbial cells that have, in turn, become a multicellular, cooperative community. Microbes, either freely living or a member of a labile, dynamic community such as a biofilm or a community within the GI tract, are enterprising, versatile forebears. Lewis Thomas, physician and writer, offered a collection of essays titled *The Lives of the Cell* in 1974.[80] He expressed in lyrical prose the vast and diverse landscape spawned by the appearance of cells on this planet. My wonderment upon viewing the dynamic life in pond water in high school was echoed in the meditative writing of this gifted essayist.

I will close this chapter by noting the obvious point that one of the constant features of life on this planet has been stress. Microbes become stressed and can counter with an elaborate, multi-component structure called a "stressosome," a usually short-lived response found in many microbial species. In the bacterium *Bacillus subtilis,* a conserved core structure is formed, from which sensory extensions are thought to specifically respond to stressors from a multitude of sources, from particles as small as photons to macromolecules. The sensory information feeds to the hub or core where these signals are thought to be integrated to activate stress-response genes, resulting in a coordinated response.[81]

In the next chapter I will focus on stress, which fuels anxiety and depression. I will also integrate learning and memory into the broader frame of stress and fear. For this chapter I will rely heavily upon studies carried out in mice. Many of these studies are published in the most highly regarded scientific journals. Investigations can be performed in mice which are not feasible for technical and ethical reasons in organisms more closely related to humans on the evolutionary scale. Nonetheless, there is a deep biological commonality between mice and humans, as has been noted, which make these studies relevant to the human condition.

CHAPTER THREE

Learning and Memory
Anxiety and Depression

THE LAST CHAPTER WAS INTENDED to convey the foundational nature of microbial complexity, facilitating an understanding of the (admittedly large) evolutionary transition from microbes to mice, an organism with the ability to memorize and learn. These traits, utilized to successfully confront a demanding existence, also bring in their wake a number of behaviors which model common human maladies, anxiety and depression, outcomes of the stresses of living.

The lively progress made in our understanding of gene function and disease mechanisms in humans is due, in no small measure, to the ascent of the mouse as model research animal.[1] While most of us would not regard the mouse as particularly endearing, scientists have nonetheless accorded this species an unquestionably elevated status. I am squarely in this camp. My research with mice in medical school revealed to me the stark picture of the "stress response." When involved in the arena of murine gene targeting as a medical school faculty, I developed an increasing appreciation for the depth of knowledge to be gained by this approach.

In times past, mouse fanciers also prized this species. They bred mice to obtain visually pleasing coat colors or unusual behaviors, exemplified by "waltzing" mice, displaying head tossing and circling behavior, later shown to be due to a degenerative process in the middle ear. Breeding "fancy" mice began as early as 80 BC in Japan.[2] These mice were transported to Europe where enthusiasts bred subspecies from the East and Europe to produce appealing specimens. The allure spread to America in the early 1890s. A retired American schoolteacher, Miss Abbie Lathrop, developed an abiding interest in these mice. She established a farm in Massachusetts to breed and sell her mice, eventually numbering more than 11,000 on her property.

Karen Rader has chronicled the early history of the murine rise to research prominence.[3] This included the efforts of Harvard's William Castle to study the genetics of coat color in these fancy mice shortly after the rediscovery of Mendel's laws in 1900, laws delineating recessive and dominant inheritance in the appearance of garden peas. A student of Castle, C. C. Little, recognized the value of inbred strains of mice to biomedical science.[4] Each inbred strain, obtained by many generations of brother-sister matings, is genetically identical. As a result, any genetic change to be studied, whether arising spontaneously in an egg or sperm or the result of a planned genetic modification, can be accomplished on a background with no genetic variation to complicate or confuse the results. The first inbred strain was derived in 1909.

Later in his life C. C. Little founded the Jackson Laboratory (known as JAX) in Bar Harbor, Maine. The importance of JAX to the research community was noted in the personal narrative. For many decades this laboratory has carried out vanguard research and established worldwide distribution of valuable, genetically engineered murine models. Investigators send their mice to JAX for distribution and "safekeeping." Embryos and/or sperm can be frozen for later re-animation when the need arises. JAX expends great effort to preserve valuable murine lines. Baylor College of Medicine is one of the centers with a large colony of these lines. When Tropical Storm Allison struck Houston in 2001 and flooded the mouse facility, JAX mounted a rescue effort to preserve these mice, as they did for institutions in the New York City area lashed by Hurricane Sandy in 2012. As I write this in 2020, the U.S is ravaged by a global pandemic caused by severe acute respiratory syndrome 2 (SARS-CoV-2), also called COVID-19. Because of threats to their workers, many facilities are curtailing their research activities, leaving murine colonies without sufficient personnel. Trucks from JAX have been sent to retrieve breeding pairs of mice to freeze embryos and sperm from these valuable models. A portion of all samples to be frozen at the laboratory in Bar Harbor are sent to another site as a hedge against future disasters. JAX provides a repository somewhat analogous to the Svalbard Global Seed Vault, where the valuable seed varieties are shielded from possible harm on a remote Norwegian island.

During the SARS-CoV-2 pandemic, immense effort is being directed toward development of an effective vaccine. Animal models, particularly mice, are key resources. Important coronavirus murine models have been developed by Stanley Perlman and Paul McCray at the medical school in Iowa City. There are many coronavirus strains which have caused epidemics. One of these was SARS-CoV, closely related to the viral pathogen causing SARS-CoV-2. Investigators noted that mice could not be infected by SARS-CoV because the virus did not attach to the murine receptor on lung surfaces. Therefore, the Iowa team produced a "transgenic" mouse in 2007 by injecting embryos with a version of the gene more closely resembling the human receptor to which the coronavirus attached with its spike proteins. The "humanized" receptor, targeted to the lung, allowed attachment of the virus and the production of lethal infection in the mice.[5] JAX requested access to this mouse model for distribution. Though live animals with the genetic modification were no longer maintained, vials of frozen sperm were shipped to JAX. This laboratory rapidly performed IVF to generate 1200 mouse pups for breeding purposes. In response to large demand, JAX has distributed this model to investigators in a frenzied attempt to obtain an effective vaccine, but also to learn more about the multi-system diseases caused by SARS-CoV and SARS-CoV-2.

Multiple advantages accrue to the mouse as a research model; short gestation (about 21 days), relatively low housing and maintenance costs, and a physiology similar to that of humans. Because of the utility of the species, megaprojects impacting human studies have received priority. Some are completed; many are ongoing. Sequencing the mouse genome was a major accomplishment,[6] completed within a short time following the published human genome sequence in 2001.[7, 8] Mice and humans shared a common ancestor approximately 75 million years ago, relatively recently measured on evolution's time scale. It should, therefore, not be a surprise that the two species have roughly the same number of genes (about 23,000), with similar genome organization. If an investigator desires to understand the function of a human gene by, for instance, inactivating the cognate gene in the mouse, there is about a 99 percent chance the murine version of that gene can be "fished out" and targeted for inactivation.

It was initially surprising that the number of genes was that low in humans. Given the complexity of our species, many scientists speculated the number would be larger, perhaps in the 100,000 range. It was likewise surprising to learn that only about 2 percent of the roughly three billion base pairs in humans encode the instructions to produce proteins. Much of the genome currently has no ascribed function. Other regions of the genome contain regulatory DNA sequences which control gene activity, determining whether the gene is "off" or "on." During embryological development, these regions are critically important in establishing the timing and tissue-specificity of "gene off" or "gene on" to reliably sculpt tissues and endow their function. The murine genome also has these regulatory regions. The exquisite regulation of genes is the bedrock for the integration of myriad pathways sustaining life; immune, endocrine, neural, metabolic, and more. It was suggested as early as 1975 that a reason humans and chimpanzees were so unlike, despite the sameness of their proteins and other macromolecules, was a differential in the manner the genes were regulated in the two species.[9] Regulatory regions figure prominently in the science to be discussed in this chapter. When a gene is targeted to a selected population of cells, regulatory DNA elements must be incorporated to permit cell specific functioning of that gene.

Having the genomes of mice and humans readily accessible—and now those of many more model organisms—has fostered the explosive growth of murine models with designed genetic modifications. The sheer volume of useful information has exponentially expanded as megaprojects have been completed. Two such projects have emanated from the Allen Institute, a joining of the Allen Institute for Brain Science and Allen Institute for Cell Science in 2015. Paul Allen, who died in 2018, was cofounder with Bill Gates of Microsoft. His interests and vision were multifaceted, as were the causes he championed.

Genes, as previously implied, are differentially expressed in different organs, and within subregions or cell populations in the same organ. In 2006 the Allen Institute produced a region-specific pattern of genes active in the murine brain at cellular resolution in a 3D format.[10, 11] Approximately two-thirds of murine genes are expressed in the brain. The major subdivisions of the mouse brain are conserved in the human brain, though the outer covering, the cortex, is much more elaborately structured, and hence complex, in humans.

In addition to gene expression data, another Allen Institute resource mined from the mouse brain is a comprehensive 3D atlas of regions and subregions of this organ, providing investigators a wealth of freely available visual information upon which to plan or assess their research.[12] This atlas was based on an amalgam of MRI (magnetic resonance imaging), gene expression data, fiber/neural tract tracing, and cell architecture delineated by multiple tissue stains.

As innovative and useful as these resources from the Allen Institute have been, another breakthrough has rendered the murine brain accessible to even more detailed observation and study. Karl Deisseroth and colleagues have developed a method termed CLARITY to render the nerve fibers of the murine brain optically transparent and permeable to reagents to study the molecular details of nerve function. This is accomplished by removal of the brain lipids through a hydrogel-based method, leaving a scaffold to support the visible nerve tracts.[13]

In addition to its service role, JAX scientists have launched many investigator-initiated projects. Loss of muscle mass and bone in conditions of microgravity is a major impediment to human long-distance space travel. Mice have been ferried to the International Space Station to study this issue.[14] Perhaps no example speaks more clearly to the utility of mice than co-clinical trials involving mice and humans. The mouse "hospital" at the Dana-Farber Institute in Boston has all the diagnostic, therapeutic, and medical imaging capacity afforded human patients, with 24-hour nursing staff. Results in mice can be translated to humans.[15] Though findings in mice do not always replicate findings in humans, these co-clinical trials speak to the commonality of the two species and are helping to foster personalized medicine.

Science is becoming more collaborative and global, with a greater emphasis on data and resource sharing. Some of this is driven by funding agencies, some by the scale required of the research effort. These welcome trends are on full display when considering the global research efforts directed toward the mouse. The NIH, along with partners in Europe, Japan, and elsewhere, have initiated a project called KOMP2—Knockout Mouse Production and Phenotyping. The goal has been to inactivate the entirety of genes in mice, one gene at a time, and to obtain phenotypes—the observable characteristics of these gene-targeted animals. The phenotype includes behavioral testing as well as a vast array of physiological parameters. JAX has been pivotal in the design and implementation of these massive undertakings.

This background on the role of mice in biomedicine leads me to a discussion of memory and learning and how these traits can dovetail into a consideration of anxiety and depression. The foregoing paragraphs have emphasized, in a large sense, that mice can be worthy surrogates in our attempts to understand human maladies. Might it be a stretch to assert we can begin to understand states of mind as complex as anxiety and depression by studying mice? All species have been challenged by environmental factors and have developed defenses and adaptations as a result. Mice, of course, are no exception. What is significant is that murine responses to challenge have familiar biological signatures which have been uncovered in exceptional detail by recent investigations.

Prior to these discussions, I return briefly to a childhood period when learning and memory were subverted. As I noted in the personal narrative, my near total mental absence in the classroom in the third grade precluded any opportunity to learn, coincident with survival of only a single, saliently negative memory. School age children have anxiety and depression, and these may have been factors, though these labels were not attached to children at that time. I think an interest in learning and memory was fueled, at least in part, by this experience.

There are two basic types of memory in humans; explicit or declarative memory which refers to conscious recall of episodes, facts, and concepts, and implicit memory which is unconscious. Riding a bicycle after learning this skill is an unconscious, procedural (implicit) memory. The locus of declarative memory formation is the hippocampus in the temporal lobes of mice and humans. At the cellular level, the pyramidal neuron within the hippocampus has been the model cell for illustrating the molecular changes underlying learning and memory. Only a few highlights from the abundant history of memory, and the neurobiological insights its study has provided, will be related here.

One patient, famous in the annals of memory, was known in life by his initials, H. M. Henry Molaison, now deceased, had severe, intractable epilepsy. His seizures originated within excitable cells in the hippocampus. No therapy had been effective. In his late 20s he underwent a partial lobectomy, resection of the middle portion of both temporal lobes, which included the hippocampus. Thereafter his seizures abated, but he was unable to form new memories.[16] Memories of his life prior to the surgery were retrievable. Many investigators who studied H. M. noted that he remained a compliant, pleasant research subject throughout the remainder of his life, existing in a "continuous present." Several books have been written about H. M., including by the grandson of the neurosurgeon who performed the operation in 1953.[17] This well-respected surgeon carried out, in addition, many so-called psychosurgeries during this era, lobectomies, a crude attempt to treat psychiatric maladies.

Eric Kandel has been a leading figure in the field, delineating the process of memory formation in the hippocampus, with subsequent transfer to regions of the cortex as the memory is consolidated. His book, *In Search of Memory*, is a compelling account of fleeing with his family from Nazi persecution of Jewish citizens of Vienna, Austria, to his desire to become a psychoanalyst and find the areas of the brain devoted to the id, ego, and superego, and ultimately to his career as psychiatrist/neuroscientist studying basic mechanisms of memory formation.[18] He was awarded a Nobel Prize in 2000 for his work. The Nobel Committee emphasized his role in demonstrating that changes in synaptic strength, emblematic of plasticity at the point one neuron joins another, were essential for memory and learning. This strengthening is termed long-term potentiation (LTP).[19] The studies Kandel and his colleagues conducted have contributed substantially to the concept of changeability in the nervous system. Experience drives change through differential gene expression at the synapse and alterations in synaptic structure. These alterations result in an increase in the number of neuronal outgrowths and synaptic connections on existing neurons. Plasticity is reliant upon these changes.[20]

Kandel and his colleagues began studying memory in *Aplysia californica*, the giant marine snail. He set out to determine if this invertebrate displayed the three forms of implicit learning that had been demonstrated in mammals; sensitization—after receiving an aversive or noxious stimulus the animal will respond to all stimuli, even benign stimuli, in an exaggerated fashion; habituation—if, after sensitization, the benign stimulus is repeatedly administered in the absence of the aversive stimulus, the animal will cease responding; and classical conditioning whereby an aversive stimulus is paired with a benign stimulus, resulting in the animal subsequently responding to the benign stimulus as strongly in the absence of the aversive stimulus as it did during the pairing. Could these be replicated in *Aplysia*?

Kandel showed that these three forms of memory can be demonstrated in *Aplysia*.[18] He concentrated on a simple reflex, the gill withdrawal reflex, controlled by neurons in an abdominal ganglion. The gill is an external organ for breathing, covered by a thin sheet called the mantle shelf, ending in the siphon. Lightly touching the siphon elicits the gill reflex, a withdrawal of the gill into the mantle cavity, a defensive mechanism to protect this delicate structure. Kandel showed that even this simple reflex can be modified by sensitization, habituation, and classical conditioning. Classical conditioning will figure prominently in discussing fear/anxiety in mice. Kandel and colleagues also showed that short-term and long-term memory could be demonstrated in this invertebrate system, anticipating studies in vertebrates revealing the processes of memory formation (short-term) and memory consolidation (long-term). In contrast to short-term memory, the conversion of memories to long-term storage or consolidation requires new protein synthesis.[21]

Kandel's work was also reductionist. He applied the knowledge he learned from the intact animal, as described, to the cellular level. He could recapitulate the three types of learning/memory in neurons from an abdominal ganglion responsible for the gill withdrawal reflex in *Aplysia*. An influential review as early as 1968 by Kandel and Alden Spencer lent credence to the value of research at the cellular level to an understanding of learning.[22] There is a hint in these and related studies of the cellular autonomy bequeathed by microbes. Reductionist approaches have been fruitful in science. A major goal is to ultimately comprehend at the systems level; systems can be understood over time by piecing together the results of painstaking, reductionist investigation.

Short-term memory, long-term memory, and LTP were demonstrated in *Aplysia*, as stated. The molecular machinery facilitating these processes have been conserved across species, from *Aplysia* and flies[23] to mammals.[18, 21] When the techniques of gene targeting, pioneered by Oliver Smithies and Mario Capecchi, became available in the late 1980s (see personal narrative), Kandel and co-workers realized the potential to utilize this technology to study synaptic plasticity in the mouse,[18] a mammal with hippocampal anatomy and function like that in humans. Mice also form explicit memories of places, objects, and other mice. In a short period of time, gene targeting, designed to inactivate a gene in the mouse, had made a major impact on the fields of immunology, development, and others, but not in a field as daunting as learning and memory. However, this began to change in the early 1990s.

In addition to Kandel, another luminary in the memory research arena is Susumu Tonegawa. He was an immunologist prior to changing his focus to neuroscience. Tonegawa was awarded a Nobel Prize in 1987 for determining the mechanisms within the adaptive immune system for creating antibody diversity, a remarkable process requiring dynamic genome rearrangement. The Kandel and Tonegawa laboratories pursued the inactivation of genes involved in LTP.[24, 25] Mice with a knock-out (KO) of these specific genes displayed defects in spatial learning. Mice are reluctant swimmers, and when immersed in a 120-centimeter cylinder of opaque water with a barely submerged platform, the mice will find and climb upon the platform. On a subsequent trial they will more quickly locate the platform, representing safety, using visual aids along the cylinder walls they had learned when initially locating the platform. The mice missing a gene involved in LTP had trouble initially locating the platform, and could not use a spatial "neural map," as did the intact control mice, to guide them in relocating the platform. These studies were the first to establish a direct link between LTP and learning. The results were met with great enthusiasm within the neuroscience community.

In the studies cited in the preceding paragraph, all the cells in the animal's body carried the inactivated gene. The mice were, however, ostensibly normal except for the learning deficit which was elicited. The concern, however, was that the KO might have produced subtle defects during development which could influence the results. Therefore, a collaboration between the Tonegawa and Kandel labs employed a technological advance, now widely utilized, to inactivate a gene exclusively in a population of hippocampal cells, the pyramidal cells, involved in memory. This would obviate the concerns expressed above. Through additional creative genetic engineering, these genes could be turned on and off at the time of the investigators' choosing, a process called conditional targeting. The two investigators conditionally inactivated a neuronal receptor known to be involved in LTP in the restricted cell population.[26] At the cellular level, LTP did not occur in pyramidal cell neurons when the gene was rendered "off." In the submerged platform test the mice were incapable of acquiring spatial information when the gene was temporarily disabled, but capable of acquiring and utilizing this information when the gene was again rendered functional.[27]

I vividly recall the time Kandel came to the medical school in Iowa City to give a talk. This energetic man with a ready, wide grin and infectious laugh brought a distinct clarity to an area of science many had considered arcane and, for the faint of heart, impracticable to approach experimentally. Kandel, in addition, has continued to write about psychiatry and pursue areas of neuroscience which have bolstered the biological foundations of this discipline.[28, 29] In medical school he planned to become a psychoanalyst. He indicated that when he undertook psychoanalysis it had been helpful.[18 (p. 182)] In the course of his career he has, however, come to the view that the rich, subtle, nuanced picture of the mind portrayed by psychoanalysts would benefit if psychiatric conditions were evaluated at the cellular/molecular level, which is increasingly being accomplished.

As I have related, I was urged to undergo psychoanalysis in medical school, not by choice, though with the hope I could become adept at free association, bringing memories, dream sequences, and snippets of everyday events to the task, striving toward insight, altered relationships, and contentment. However, finding that submerged platform of psychological insights with the compromised mental/emotional tools I possessed, deficient in the ability to form a "neural map" to navigate toward these elevated ideals, was beyond achievement for the closed person I was at that time. Memory, the wellspring of so much of our emotional lives, is a sublime trait.

⸭

AN IMPRESSIVE development in the quest to interrogate the deeper levels of neuronal function in rodents has been that of optogenetics, as noted in the personal narrative. Optogenetics is the creative merging of the molecules of vision with the increasing ability to target genes carried by viruses to selected cell populations within a specified region of the brain, genes which encode these vision molecules. A third component of optogenetics is the capacity to direct a light source onto these light-responsive proteins to either activate or inhibit neurons and neural tracts which mediate the functions of the brain. The ancient and large class of genes which have enabled these studies, the opsin genes, are derived from microorganisms such as algae and archaea. If neuronal activation is the goal, the protein encoded by an opsin gene transduces one form of energy, light, into another form, electrical current, the means of neural communication. If inhibition is the goal, light is focused on an opsin which causes the neuronal membrane to become more resistant to "firing." Blue light targeted to a designated opsin is activating, whereas yellow light on a different opsin is inhibitory. Other selected characteristics of the manner by which light is administered is key to experimental success.

⁞⁞⁞

BEFORE DISCUSSING the utility of optogenetics, a brief "primer" on neurotransmission may assist this effort. For those interested, the history of this subject is riveting,[30] the discovery that neurotransmission relies upon chemicals *and* electrical transmission, the "soups and sparks." Sprouting from the surface of neurons are dendrites. The "upstream" neuron sends its single axon to make connections with these dendrites at the synapse, the cleft across which the neural message is communicated from the presynaptic to the postsynaptic terminal via a neurotransmitter. An action potential is triggered when the summation of activity at these connections reaches a threshold, provoking movement of sodium and potassium ions across the cell membrane. The amino acid glutamate is the primary neurotransmitter at excitatory synapses, accounting for about 50 per cent of transmission. The primary inhibitory neurons are called interneurons; the majority of these cells utilize the neurotransmitter GABA (gamma-aminobutyric acid). In addition to many classes of neurotransmitters, another category of chemical agents which affect neural function, and hence behavior, are the neuro-modulators. These typically bind to cell surface receptors and are taken into the cell where they initiate a cascade of signaling molecules. There are multiple neuromodulators, including dopamine, serotonin, acetylcholine, norepinephrine, and others, including hormones like cortisol released into the blood stream. Neuromodulators are widely expressed in the brain.

Another feature of coherent brain activity which impinges optogenet-ics is rhythmicity.[31] Neural networks oscillate at different frequencies in rhythmic fashion. Neural activity is often modulated by a rhythm called the theta rhythm. The settings chosen to administer light to the opsin genes to activate or inhibit neural activity are informed by known rhythmic activity of regions of the brain. The hippocampus is a key region which has influenced the understanding of brain rhythms.

The person largely responsible for bringing the elements of optoge-netics together in a freely behaving mouse is Karl Deisseroth, previously mentioned for his invention of CLARITY. Accomplishing each of the three converging aspects of optogenetics was individually a major feat.[32] On the role of opsins in revealing fine details of cellular function Deisseroth says, evoking the origin of mitochondria, "....microbial DNA has yet again returned to eukaryotic cells, a recurrent and curious theme of life on earth over billions of years, to provide another symbiosis, this one scientific. Such relationships coevolve and persist once formed, and though biology in the coming years will continue to move in unexpected directions, the ancient microbial opsins now seem inextricably part of our journey."[32 (p. 1224)] Deisseroth is a psychiatrist and neuroscientist whose goal, like Kandel's, is to erect a basic science foundation undergirding psychiatry.

Bioluminescence is widespread in nature. This colorful display, the absorption and emission of light, has been harnessed to observe cellular activity as it happens. An early indication of how valuable the suite of light-emitting proteins was to become was heralded by the isolation of GFP, green fluorescent protein, from jellyfish. This was accomplished after years of work by Osamu Shimomura. When GFP absorbs light in the blue wavelength spectrum, it emits a green fluorescence. Martin Chalfie's group reported the incorporation of GFP into bacteria and round worms in 1994.[33] Soon thereafter Roger Tsien and colleagues modified the chemical structure of GFP in multiple ways to produce fluorescence of many colors,[34] allowing different, functionally distinct cells to be visualized in living animals. When Tsien died following an accident, he was working productively on several major questions, including the storage of long-term memories. Based on his work, tissues can now be rendered a "rainbow" of colors under the microscope. The three investigators cited in this paragraph won Nobel Prizes in 2008 for their GFP investigations.

Optogenetics, building upon the earlier work in bioluminescence, has had a major impact on memory research. Memories which are stored are referred to as engrams, a term Richard Semon articulated in the early twentieth-century to describe a collection of cells, "engram cells," which he hypothesized undergo basic physiochemical changes elicited by learning. An engram approximates a "memory trace." Josselyn and Tonegawa have recently summarized the extensive literature on engram studies,[35] revealing the sophisticated technologies, principally optogenetics, which have allowed us to "see" memories in the making and their fate as they are stored (consolidated), recalled, and reconsolidated.

As an interesting aside, neuronal competition and selection drive memory formation. Many processes in biological systems are subject to Darwinian competition, implying that selection partitions "winners" and "losers." A prime example of a competitive process is the development of the brain. More brain-forming neural progenitors are produced than will be incorporated into the brain; many are "pruned" via a competitive process. The neurons selected to participate in an engram are those which are most excitable or electrically active at the time of memory formation. A surrogate for this activity is a molecule called CREB,[36] also found to play a key role in memory in Kandel's studies of *Aplysia*. Those neurons with higher levels of CREB are more excitable, and hence more plastic.[37] As Kandel and others have revealed, it is this plasticity which is the hallmark of learning and memory.

The memory studies cited throughout this section are invariably reliant upon production of fear memories in rodents, usually mice, but rats have also contributed. There has been no testing paradigm which has been as informative in delineating memory pathways as the creation of a fear memory in mice. The outward physical manifestation of fear and its recall is "freezing," an innate response to a conditioning regimen, as described below, and to other inciting stimuli. Freezing is observed in species from flies to primates in response to fear-provoking situations. Sustained fear promotes anxiety in mice and humans. Anxiety-like behavior can be assessed in mice, as will also be described.

The use of the term anxiety in relation to murine behavior is validated by myriad studies showing anxious states involve similar brain regions in mice and humans. The experiments in mice are made more challenging, of course, by the inability of mice to verbalize their symptoms. In addition to brain imaging studies in humans, mice and humans respond similarly to drugs which act upon pathways mediating fear and anxiety.

Inducing fear memories takes advantage of Pavlovian conditioning, also called classical conditioning. Pavlov demonstrated that the pairing of a neutral stimulus such as a bell ring (the conditioned stimulus) with a potent stimulus, food (the unconditioned stimulus), causes a dog to salivate when the neutral stimulus is presented in the absence of food. A similar associative learning process occurs in the minds of mice when a conditioned stimulus, such as a loud noise, is paired with an aversive stimulus, usually a mild foot shock (unconditioned stimulus). Alternatively, a mouse may be placed in an unfamiliar cage, which is then paired with a foot shock. After as few as one or several such pairings, a return to this cage will elicit a similar reaction, freezing. This is called context fear conditioning. A control animal placed in an unfamiliar cage without the shock will not freeze when reintroduced to the cage. Fear learning and its expression, as noted, provides us with the best understood, most fruitful neurobehavioral model of learning and memory. With meticulous precision, the neural circuits underlying fear and its consequences are being "teased out" in a fashion that provides a time course and anatomic specificity which did not exist prior to optogenetics.

Numerous measures will betray whether an experimental manipulation is anxiety inducing—anxiogenic—or anxiety relieving—anxiolytic—compared to controls, mice which have not undergone any form of conditioning. The most frequently employed tests for anxiety in mice are the open field test and the elevated maze plus test, though other testing schemes are available.[38] In the open field test, mice are placed into a brightly lit enclosure to which they have had no previous exposure. Anxiety-like behavior is assessed by documenting the time spent along the less well-lit walls, avoiding the center. In the elevated plus maze, an elevated platform supports two intersecting, enclosed arms, one darkened and the other brightly lit. An anxious mouse spends more time in the darkened arm, with fewer forays into the lit arm.

The neural landscape of fear and anxiety consists of, but is clearly not limited to, three principal brain structures/regions; the amygdala, the hippocampus, and the prefrontal cortex,[39] an area involved in cognition and planning. The medial portion of the prefrontal cortex is reciprocally linked to the basolateral portion of the amygdala, the structure critical in the initial stages of fear memory formation. Fear memories are formed and extinguished over time. The prefrontal cortex plays a major role in both processes.[40]

The amygdala is a particularly intriguing structure, implicated in emotional and social behaviors, particularly those related to fear, anxiety, and aggression. Every vertebrate species has an amygdala. Even reptiles, birds, and fish have an amygdala-like structure with connections and functions like those in mammals. The amygdala is not only involved in responding to negative or aversive stimuli, but also to positive stimuli. Thus, its role in determining valence, good or bad, is critical in finding food and mates, and avoiding danger. Joseph LeDoux has studied the amygdala for many years[41] and is among a cadre of neuroscientists that have revealed the roles of this brain region in our emotional lives. The amygdala is composed of regions and subregions with many types of neurons. The basolateral complex and the central nucleus figure most prominently in the subject under discussion. The central nucleus, like the basolateral complex, is composed of subregions with multiple neuronal subtypes.

The fear pathways we have been describing begin within the amygdala. Sensory information, such as an auditory tone, is processed in other brain regions and is transferred to the basolateral amygdala. This sensory input is integrated within the basolateral amygdala with a stimulus such as a foot shock via associative learning. This bundled package is then relayed to the central nucleus of the amygdala which has output relays to other brain structures where the behavioral/physiological effects are made manifest. The central nucleus projects to structures such as the hypothalamus which mediates the neuromodulatory portion of the fear circuit, causing release of stress hormones, cortisol in humans and corticosterone in rodents, and to the brainstem where regulatory centers elevate the heart and respiratory rates via the autonomic nervous system, mediated by epinephrine and norepinephrine. Other centers which receive central nucleus information participate in the defensive behavioral states which fear can provoke, from passive freezing to aggressive action.

Just as the patient H. M., mentioned earlier, had revealed the key role of the hippocampus in memory formation, another patient, S. M., helped to document the centrality of the amygdala in fear processing.[42] She had a rare genetic disorder, Urbach-Wiethe syndrome, which damaged her amygdalae. Apart from a selective deficit in the ability to recognize and process fear, her neuropsychological assessment was otherwise normal. She could not recognize fearful facial expressions. She could, however, verbalize the concept of fear. Though she did not feel the emotion of fear, she could experience other emotions normally.

Fear is clearly an emotionally arousing experience, leading to activation of the hypothalamus-pituitary-adrenal axis and consequent release of stress hormones. Whether positive or negative, emotion-laden memories facilitate the storage and recall of these memories.[43] If the hippocampus is the "memory center," how does the hippocampus become involved? A quote from a LeDoux paper will suffice to explain the centrality of the amygdala and involvement of the hippocampus: "In addition to its role in emotion, the amygdala is also involved in the regulation or modulation of a variety of cognitive functions, such as attention, perception, and explicit memory. It is generally thought that those functions are modulated by the amygdala; processing of the emotional significance of external stimuli. Outputs of the amygdala then lead to the release of hormones and/or neuromodulators in the brain that then alter cognitive processing in cortical areas. For example, explicit memories about emotional situations are enhanced via amygdala outputs that ultimately affect the hippocampus: glucocorticoid hormone released into the blood stream via amygdala activity travels to the brain and then binds to neurons in the basal amygdala; the latter then connects to the hippocampus to enhance explicit memory."[41] (p. R873)

Optogenetics has expanded and refined our understanding of the mechanisms and neural circuits establishing fear. As implied above, neuroscientists reasoned that neurons in the basolateral amygdala, specifically the pyramidal cells, were likely to demonstrate the plasticity required of associative fear learning. LeDoux and colleagues, including Deisseroth, sought direct confirmation in a study in rats.[44] Virus with an opsin gene targeted to basolateral amygdala pyramidal cells was injected into the region. Days later an optical source was inserted into the same region. An auditory tone was then repeatedly paired with flashes of light, activating the opsin molecules which, in turn, depolarized the neurons to initiate firing. By this means a fear memory was established, made known by the freezing behavior which occurred when the tone was presented in the absence of a light flash. Pyramidal cells had "learned" the association which set in motion the train of events which resulted in freezing.

In the rodent, as in humans, the push and pull of excitation and inhibition involving specific pathways, acting in concert with molecular signaling, determine the behavioral manifestations of fear. A hint of this complexity will be cited in a few representative studies. Even within the amygdala, opposing effects can be elicited. One of the earliest studies to demonstrate the differential sensitivity of terminal projections from the basolateral to the central nucleus of the amygdala came from the Deisseroth group.[45] Selective illumination of opsin molecules which activate these fiber tracts terminating in the central amygdala produced a rapidly reversible anxiolytic effect, whereas optogenetic inhibition increased anxiety-related behavior in the open field and elevated plus maze tests.

Further, it is possible to probe the role of the various classes of cells resident within the amygdala, some of which are interneurons which generally inhibit electrical activity of neurons. Optogenetics is a major tool, but not the only one. Pharmacologic and electrophysiologic recordings provide complementary data. In a representative study using these tools, it was demonstrated that a microcircuit of interneuron cells "gated" the downstream responses to fear conditioning emanating from the central nucleus of the amygdala.[46] A major question from studies such as this is delineation of the pathways which regulate not only the anxiety-like behavioral manifestations of an isolated episode of fear, but the causal landscape which regulates fear generalization, the development of anxiety which extends beyond fear episodes. Though MRI in humans does not have the temporal specificity nor the fine-grained anatomic detail that optogenetics provides in mice, it can reveal disordered neural connectivity in subregions of the amygdala in humans with generalized anxiety disorder.[47]

As noted repeatedly, many brain structures contribute to fear and anxiety. Another study from the Deisseroth laboratory was a fine-grained look at the differential neural pathways in a brain region called the bed nucleus of the stria terminalis (BNST). This nucleus is a key modulator of states of fear and anxiety in humans[48] and mice. The BNST is often referred to as the extended amygdala. Two subregions of the murine BNST were investigated.[49] A neural pathway in one region, when stimulated, produced a fearful, anxious state. In contrast, a neural tract in a different BNST subregion reduced anxiety when compared to control mice. Within the region mediating anxiety reduction, the authors revealed three separable pathways which, respectively, elicited three specific indices of anxiolysis. One pathway to the hypothalamus reduced the innate tendency of mice to avoid open spaces. Another pathway to the respiratory center in the brain stem reduced breathing rate. A third pathway to the region of the brain associated with dopamine, a "reward" neurotransmitter, increased positive valence, measured in a test called real-time place preference wherein a mouse could freely explore two chambers. Optogenetic activation of the pathway terminating in the dopamine region of the brain when the mouse was in one of the two chambers resulted in the mouse showing preference for that chamber.

Concurrent with many of the studies referenced above, the brains of these mice have been sectioned to microscopically display the cellular anatomy made vivid by the distinguishing colors. Further molecular studies can be accomplished as well as an assessment of electrical activity of the neural tracts exposed in the sections. Electrophysiologic investigations of these tracts may supplement those which can be performed in freely behaving mice. Through optogenetic, molecular, and electrical studies, Kandel, Tonegawa, Deisseroth, and many others have revealed numerous, shrouded aspects of learning and memory, and in the process opened a window onto one of the most vexing infirmities which afflicts humankind, anxiety.

Anxiety is more encompassing than the emotion of fear. Anxiety disorders include phobias, generalized anxiety disorder, panic disorder, and post-traumatic stress disorder (PTSD). The diagnosis of PTSD, taken verbatim,[50] requires that a person was exposed to a traumatic event or an extreme stressor to which he/she responded with fear, helplessness or horror; further, that the person exhibit three types of symptoms; reexperiencing the event, avoidance of reminders of the event, and hyperarousal for at least a month. Hyperarousal causes irritability, insomnia, poor concentration, hypervigilance, and increased startle reaction. PTSD shares symptoms with, and increases the risk for, generalized anxiety disorder, panic disorder, major depression, and substance abuse.

PTSD is powerfully influenced by memory. One means to overcome PTSD is via extinction training, recalling and facing one's fears to attempt to eliminate the fear memory. Even if there appears to be initial success, fear memories may spontaneously reappear. The engrams representing fear memories are distinct from the neurons selected for extinction of a fear memory. Thus, new learning is required for extinction. Methods described in this chapter allow investigators to "tag" neurons which constitute a fear memory and those for extinguishing a fear memory or engram in mice. Using optogenetics, these neuron populations can be either activated or inhibited in mice.[51] Basic studies such as these can be a gateway to finding enduring remedies for PTSD. In addition to PTSD, other disorders which can be studied in mice by optogenetics include autism, addiction, Parkinson disease, and epilepsy.

The foregoing offers just a glimpse of the complexity underlying the genesis of fear and anxiety in a mammal. Fear is an evolutionarily old and preserved protective mechanism. Neural circuits which scan the environment for threats and initiate defensive reactions are modified by fear. This "survival circuit" can become dysfunctional if it continues to be engaged in the absence of external or internal threat, leading to diffuse, persisting apprehension and wariness, a state of anxiety.

⁂

I UNDERTOOK this writing, in part, to learn more about these mental states which have had a profound personal effect and deeply impacted the lives of persons I was close to (Chapter 1). Depression and anxiety are often co-mingled. I believe I experienced these two states in approximately equal measure. I further believe that a component of the anxiety I experienced was induced by the uncertainty, bewilderment, and mystery of what I was feeling and the apprehension about how and when, pray God, this would end? The dysphoria accompanying the depression was at its worst in medical school. The intrusion of suicidal ideation, though without a plan or serious intent, was distressing in the extreme. For variable periods of time this was associated with an anxiety that one day suicide would become an inevitability.

Optogenetics and other tools mentioned previously have not elucidated depression to the extent it has for anxiety. This disorder has not yielded a physiological correlate as accessible and informative as a fear memory. Nonetheless, optogenetics has been a valuable tool. There are common biological underpinnings which link many psychiatric conditions; anxiety and depression, as previously noted, frequently co-exist.[52] It might be expected that neural and molecular pathways underlying both conditions engage common brain regions. This is, indeed, the case.

How can an investigator ascertain depression in a rodent? Though most of the optogenetic studies and testing schemes involve mice, rats react to stress in a similar manner. Two tests used as rapid screens for depression-like behavior in the mouse are the forced swim and tail suspension tests. A mouse placed in a small cylinder of water will attempt to escape. It has been largely accepted (though there are skeptics) that a depressed mouse will cease effortful movements sooner than a control mouse. Similarly, a depressed mouse suspended by the tail will stop escape-related struggles and hang limp sooner than a mouse which has not undergone stressful encounters. This has been dubbed "behavioral despair."

If a mouse shows behavioral despair, other, more elaborate testing is utilized which includes acute stress, but more commonly mild, chronic stress is employed from which there is no escape during the conditioning phase. An example would include unpredictable, twice a day stresses such as mild foot shock over 10 days. The depressed mouse, when later returned to the cage where the stress occurred but now provided an escape route, does not attempt to escape. This has been categorized as "learned helplessness," a passive response to the previously imposed circumstances. Further, animals can be subjected to bullying by placing them in a cage daily for a brief period for 10 days with an aggressive, larger mouse from a different inbred strain. At the end of this daily encounter, the bullied mouse is returned to its home cage, though always in view of the aggressor. This produces behavior characterized as "social defeat," manifested as lessened social interaction with non-bullying mice. Humans with depression lose the ability to experience pleasure, known as anhedonia. Mice mimic this by losing their preference for sucrose-sweetened drinking water. Further validity accrues to these models of depressive behavior in the many studies in which antidepressant medications (usually the selective serotonin reuptake inhibitor Prozac) ameliorates the observed depressive behavior. As with anxiety, the pathways shown to be operative in murine models are also implicated in human functional magnetic resonance imaging (fMRI) studies.

When discussing anxiety, I selected a small sampling of the available literature. This will, likewise, be the case for depression. The articles cited will primarily be those utilizing optogenetics. It is important to reiterate that learning and memory are facilitated by plasticity within the central nervous system; depression and anxiety insinuate into this changeable matrix of neural tissue. The complex gene-environment interactions impacting depressed and anxious individuals drive this plasticity in specific circuits, pathways which are increasingly amenable to investigation. As stated, brain structures implicated in anxiety, the amygdala, hippocampus, and prefrontal cortex, are also prominent fixtures on the landscape of depression. As with anxiety, multiple other structures contribute to the neural cascades of depression. Regions which are more specific to depression vs anxiety, such as the ventral tegmental area (VTA) and nucleus accumbens (NAc), among others, will receive mention.

Depression is highly individual and heterogeneous in its causation, producing a range of symptoms—depressed mood, psychomotor retardation or agitation, reduced motivation, hopelessness, suicidality, and anhedonia. Major contenders for the pathogenesis of depression include alterations in the signaling of neurotransmitters and neuromodulators, primarily serotonin, norepinephrine, and dopamine; deficits in brain reward processes impacting dopamine pathways; abnormal neurogenesis (new nerve cell generation) in the hippocampus.[53] Many or all these factors may overlap and become expressed to a greater or lesser extent. Another factor, abnormal cognitive styles exemplified by negative thinking, cannot be modeled in nonverbal species.[54]

The brain's reward pathway is implicated in mood disorders. The principal reward pathway extends from the ventral tegmental area (VTA), the location of dopamine-containing neurons, to the nucleus accumbens (NAc) in the forebrain. In the past this pathway has been primarily implicated in addiction, with its role in depression and social phobias a more recent focus. Responses to reward are mediated by many of the same brain regions which, in different (stressful) contexts, produce depressive behaviors. The evolutionary drive to seek reward is strong in addiction, though weak in the setting of depression.

Utilizing light-induced activation of an opsin targeted to the basolateral amygdala-NAc tract, investigators revealed a pathway which signaled through one type of dopamine receptor to promote reward seeking.[55] Direct proof that the dopamine-mediated reward pathways also regulate depressive behaviors was provided by optogenetics and the behavioral assays which have been developed.[56] Opsins had been microinjected that would inhibit or activate dopamine neurons in the VTA. Light-induced inhibition produced a significant reduction in sucrose preference and increased behavioral despair, evidenced by decreased efforts when suspended by the tail or placed in the swimming cylinder. Activation of these neurons projecting to the NAc rapidly reversed these effects. Additionally, anhedonia was also produced by chronic, mild stress, as was learned helplessness when the rodents were conditioned to inescapable stress. As with behavioral despair, these effects were also reversed upon activation of the pathway. The conclusions were bolstered using electrophysiologic evaluation and pharmacological agents. In a related study, the VTA-NAc pathway and the VTA-medial prefrontal cortex pathways showed opposing effects in mice expressing anhedonia.[57] Optogenetics permits an investigation of other pathways which project to and exit from the VTA which can exert opposing influences, either reward or aversion.[58]

A pathway from the hippocampus to the NAc was also shown to regulate reward behavior via the strength of the hippocampus-NAc synapses independent of dopamine signaling. Increased electrical activity of this pathway produced LTP (long-term potentiation) which, in turn, drove preference for a cage in which the mouse had previously encountered another mouse, a positive event. This resulted in a learning process called conditioned place preference. Stress eliminated LTP and conditioned place preference.[59] This study reveals, again, the connection of LTP and plasticity, and suggests that this plasticity is key for contextual reward behavior.

An interesting study from the Tonegawa laboratory links emotional memory to depressive behavior and its relief.[60] Memory-forming neurons in the hippocampus were "tagged" with light-sensitive opsin genes as described, and the opsin protein was light-activated when the memory, or engram, was being formed. As indicated in the section on anxiety, the Tonegawa lab had previously shown that once a memory engram has been established via tagged hippocampal neurons, the memory would be recalled when light was again directed onto the same neurons. In one group this memory was formed when an individual male was put in a cage with a female, a pleasurable episode. A second group was individually placed in an empty cage, a neutral experience. A third group was subjected to immobilization restraint, an obvious negative experience. The animals in all three groups were then exposed to 10 consecutive days of stress. As a result of these conditioning regimens, the animals in all groups exhibited passivity and decreased interest in previously engaging activities. The depressive behavior was alleviated only in the mice whose activated memory recall was the encounter with a female. More extensive investigations in this study identified the hippocampus to amygdala to NAc pathways as the probable route underlying the relief from the maladaptive behavior after only a single light-activated recall. The relief was longer lasting with chronic activation of the hippocampal engram cells.

An additional important finding in this study related to the formation of new neurons, neurogenesis, a subject I will return to in the next chapter. Stressed animals showed reduced neurogenesis. Chronic activation of the engram encoding a pleasant memory not only rescued the impaired behavior induced by stress, it also normalized production of new neurons.

Another brain region, among many, influencing the development of depression is the habenula which mediates neural communication between the forebrain and structures in the midbrain. This region is active in monkeys when an aversive event is expected, or an expected reward is withheld.[61] In rats undergoing either an acute or chronic learned helplessness protocol, investigators revealed that enhanced transmission of neural activity from other brain regions onto neurons in the habenula which project to the VTA contributes to learned helplessness. Deep brain stimulation of the lateral habenula in these mice suppressed this excitatory synaptic transmission and reversed the observed helplessness.[62] In humans, deep brain stimulation to several distinct brain regions participating in depressive pathways has offered promise to a subset of patients not responding to more conventional therapies.[63] This therapy is high-frequency electrical stimulation that is milder and more targeted than electroconvulsive therapy. Much remains to be learned about how deep brain stimulation works and the location of pathways impacted by this form of therapy. Optogenetics has a role in delineating some of these issues.[64]

Though the mouse has been the primary focus for modeling diseases such as anxiety and depression for many technical and biological reasons, other models have contributed.[65] Nonhuman primates such as Rhesus monkeys reveal affective signs of depression when stressed and neural correlates can be demonstrated by fMRI, though detailed circuitry and molecular changes underlying the behaviors cannot be explored in detail for ethical reasons. Animals toward the other end of evolutionary complexity, species such as zebrafish, can also be profitably studied. An endocrine response to stress and danger is elicited in this species as characteristically as in other vertebrates. Multiple genetically engineered murine models of alterations in the hypothalamic-pituitary-adrenal axis has uncovered depressive and anxious behaviors related to specific molecular signaling within these neuromodulatory pathways. Similarly, in a zebrafish model found to have an inherited mutation in the glucocorticoid receptor leading to high levels of cortisol, the fish freeze when placed in a novel tank and cease exploratory activities.[66] Control fish do not display these behaviors in the same circumstances. These fish did not habituate, as repeated exposure to the novel tank produced the same behavior. When the zebrafish with the mutation were returned to the familiar aquarium with other fish, their behavior normalized, as it did when treated with the commonly used antidepressant Prozac. As the experiments with zebrafish attest, there is deep phylogenetic conservation of organismal reactions to stress.

The prefrontal cortex, as stated, is also integrally involved in depression-related behavior, exemplified by a study in rats.[67] The prefrontal cortex provides higher-level modulation of cognitive behavior, as well as decisions to act. Stimulation of a subset of prefrontal cortex neurons terminating in the brainstem region housing the serotonergic neurons, associated with major depression, produced motivated escape behavior in the forced swim test when the activating opsin was stimulated by light. The opposite effect was seen when a light source implanted over the lateral habenula activated a subset of neurons projecting from the prefrontal cortex to this region. This study, and others which have been referenced, highlights the critical balance of inhibitory and excitatory flow to and from multiple brain regions in the production of altered mental states.

Embedded within the neural pathways which facilitate depressive responses are the interacting molecular pathways. A major focus of stress-related studies is brain-derived neurotrophic factor (BDNF). This protein is widely expressed in the brain, including the hippocampus where it participates in learning and memory processes, as well as stimulation of new neuron growth. BDNF interacts with stress hormones; glucocorticoid signaling, in concert with BDNF, enhances the vulnerability to stress and the expression of fear memories.[68]

Susceptibility to depression is countered by resilience. What factors confer resistance to stress? While not fully known, studies in mice can provide biological measures which help answer the question. Socially defeated mice demonstrate social avoidance, an effect dependent upon BDNF and responsive to long-term antidepressants.[69] There is, however, variance in the degree of susceptibility, allowing segregation of mice deemed susceptible or resistant.[70] Chronic social defeat increased the levels of BDNF in the NAC of susceptible mice. In this study BDNF was not the only protein which showed skewed expression. Many genes were differentially regulated in the VTA and NAC when comparing the two groups of mice, an expected outcome when organismal homeostasis is perturbed.

One possibility the authors considered to explain the difference in phenotype (susceptible vs resistant) in these genetically identical mice raised under the same environmental conditions was epigenetics, defined by a heritable change in the phenotype which is not caused by an alteration in the DNA sequence. Epigenetics is one of many regulators of gene expression. Epigenetics is thought to be an important factor which influences the gene-environment interaction, allowing the integration of an animal's genome with environmental signals. It could be a major influence when genetically identical twins reared in the same household display different traits. A common epigenetic "marker" or change is the presence or absence of a methyl group on a particular nucleotide. Alterations in methylation or other epigenetic chemical changes are a means of turning genes on and off.

In the late 1990s and early 2000s, Michael Meaney and his colleagues published studies which linked maternal behavior and epigenetics in their offspring. They relied upon observations of nursing Norway rats and potential negative consequences for the development of the stress response system in their pups. The outcome was most favorable if the mothers assumed an arched-back posture with frequent licking and grooming of their young during nursing bouts. When offspring of mothers displaying low amounts of licking and grooming and altered posture became adults, these rats showed exaggerated responses to restraint stress. Their levels of corticosterone were significantly higher. These animals were more fearful than offspring of nurturing mothers. Other assays of central nervous system tissue showed evidence of a dysregulated stress response.[71]

The Meaney group then cross-fostered female pups born to low licking/grooming mothers to high licking/grooming mothers. When adults, these females were less fearful and showed high rates of licking/grooming of pups when they became nursing mothers, and vice versa.[72] This "programming" of stress reactivity occurs quickly following birth, is durable, and illustrates the transmission of behavioral traits across generations.

The same group later showed an epigenetic mark which was associated with this maternal behavior and was plausibly the causative change. The stress pathway encompasses the hippocampus, as previously noted. The investigators uncovered a difference in the methylation status of a gene which regulates the glucocorticoid receptor in the hippocampus. A methyl group was added to the glucocorticoid receptor in the first postnatal week in pups born to high licking/grooming mothers and was reversed by cross fostering the pups to low licking/grooming mothers.[73] The thread from zebrafish with a glucocorticoid receptor mutation to mice with a methylated glucocorticoid receptor is bolstered by a study associating epigenetic regulation of the glucocorticoid receptor in human postmortem brains with cases of child abuse.[74]

Epigenetics appears to be a bridge across the nature/nurture divide. The fact that phenotypes can be nongenomically altered in response to the environment potentially represents a deep reservoir of durable biological responses when organisms interact with others or encounter novel habitats. Epigenetics may even play a role in speciation.[75]

Epigenetics is a level of gene regulation above the basic DNA sequence, as noted. The reader may wonder if these are any genetic "markers" revealed by sequencing the genomes of depressed humans and comparing these sequences to those of individuals who are not depressed. Studies called GWAS, genome wide association studies, have been fruitful in revealing genes predisposing to many diseases. The attempt to do so for depression has, until recently been unrevealing. In a study of Chinese women with severe depression, two markers were found, one linked to a gene important for the structure of mitochondria, the energy producing organelle.[76] This finding is intriguing because of the known association of depression and amotivational states in many depressed individuals.

Studies with a GWAS design implicate single genes. Studies with a related design implicate regions of the genome which confer disease susceptibility, evaluating genomic stretches called haplotypes. On this topic, it is of interest that anatomically modern humans, that group that migrated out of Africa approximately 60,000 years ago, interbred with Neandertals. The genomes of modern Eurasians, as a result, contain a small fraction of DNA, between 1.5–4 percent, inherited from this group of archaic humans. Though this fraction of DNA is small, haplotypes predisposing to depression and other disorders have been inherited from Neandertals.[77]

The genetics of psychiatric illness writ large is convoluted and complex. Persons like Ken Kendler who have been at the forefront of this field have opined that we are embarking upon a new era in which molecular technologies and improved statistical methodology will permit investigators to perceive, as he puts it, "through a glass darkly," the biology which becomes disordered in these diseases.[78]

The studies cited in this chapter lend credence to the biological commonality of maladaptive states from mice to humans. Are we, therefore, ready to admit mice to the fraternity of the suffering? Despite the evidence of deep biological connections extending across time, many are not ready to privilege rodents in this manner. Considering the difficulty we have in describing personal pain, could we possibly ever know the mind of a mouse? To state the absurdly obvious, mice cannot communicate feelings of worthlessness and suicidality. But as behavioral assessments, laboratory assays, and squiggles on a chart tracking electrical activity become ever more revealing, more of us may come to a grudging acceptance of the mental struggles of our fellow beings.

We can widen and help inform this discussion of the functional links among memory, learning, anxiety, and depression through a consideration of emotion, long neglected as a topic suitable for investigation and discourse. This stance has been reconsidered. Emotions are now accorded the status of other fields of neuroscience. Emotions are often linked to pleasant thoughts. They can also become dysregulated, leading to commonly experienced mental distress. It is to this and related inquiries I next turn.

CHAPTER 4

Emotion

Inching Toward Consciousness

IN THE PREVIOUS CHAPTER I endeavored to show that neuroscientists have gained a relatively deep understanding of memory and learning, though inevitable gaps remain. Using tools such as optogenetics in rodents, I also cited a portion of the growing literature linking the neural structures subserving learning and memory to anxiety and depression. The brain areas and neuromodulatory systems that contribute to fear and anxiety overlap, not only in humans but also in animals.[1] There is also overlap between fear/ anxiety and stress/depression circuits.[2] Drugs targeted to these conditions affect the same molecular pathways implicated in learning and memory.[3] Finally, the known association between plasticity and learning and memory applies to the development—and relief—of anxiety and depression. These interrelationships are profound.

I now seek to widen the lens on anxiety and depression by yoking them to emotions. Dysregulation of emotion underlies these maladies. As also noted in the last chapter, the study of fear conditioning/learning has been a model to understand an emotion at the microcircuit level, explicating the neuroanatomical, neurochemical, and electrophysiological dimensions. This comprehension does not exist for the other emotions, discussed below.

Emotions have a powerful hold on our thinking and actions, providing a plausible entry into that elusive, ineffable trait we designate as consciousness. An adequate description of consciousness does not exist, despite centuries of debate by philosophers and scientists. At its base, it is awareness of our internal and external environment; we instinctively know it exists. Proponents of multiple different theories have gamely attempted to uncover its core features. Ongoing work may permit productive attempts to study this trait via the same scientific principles which have explained other "mysteries" such as the quantum world. Many of the authors who study and write about emotions interweave their conceptions of the link between emotion and consciousness into their publications. I will follow this thread.

Emotions are mental states which have been accorded scientific respectability only relatively recently. As mentioned, understanding the emotion of fear has shown what is possible and has been a factor which has made the study of emotions respectable. Scientists could not have been faulted for avoiding emotion research in the past; emotions were deemed to be too subjective, eclipsed in relevance by the study of cognition—perception, attention, memory—and related fields.

Though emotion research has attracted many notable investigators, no agreed upon definition has been put forward over the decades since psychologist William James asked *What is an Emotion?* in 1884.[4] Many queries are subsumed within James' question. How many emotions are there? Are there primary—or core—emotions and secondary emotions? What regions of the brain generate an emotion? Are there neural circuits dedicated to each emotion, or do they overlap? What can we say about the expression of emotion in animals? For each emotion, is there an innate, hard-wired component and an experiential or learned component? Are emotions expressed in a similar manner across disparate cultures? How do feelings relate to emotion?

Much that is imbedded within these questions is incompletely known. James has also illuminated another conundrum related to the emotion/behavior nexus; does an emotion cause the observed behavior we associate with an emotion, or does the behavior cause the emotion? James alleged we are sad because we cry, not the reverse. The emotion, in his view, is the consequence of the behavior.

Two investigators at the forefront of emotion research, Ralph Adolphs and David Anderson, argue the commonly held stance that emotions cause behavior, though concede that once a behavior is cued it can feed back to elicit further emotional content.[5] They, and others, also assert that feelings and emotions are not equivalent, but related. They define a feeling as the conscious experience of an emotion. This is similar to the assertion of Joseph LeDoux who has stated that the consciously experienced feeling *is* the emotion.[6] Antonio Damasio, who draws a distinction between feelings and emotions, nonetheless has noted that consciousness must be added for an organism to know it has a feeling.[7] One straightforward observation is that feelings apply more broadly (such as "I feel tired," etc.) than emotions.

What are the basic or primary emotions? Many authors cite Paul Ekman who studied human facial expressions in response to emotion-provoking cues across a wide range of cultures. He argued for a commonality of these responses. As a result of his observations, he proposed six universal emotions: fear, sadness, happiness, disgust, surprise, and anger.[8] Ekman's work is broadly congruent with that of Darwin who investigated emotions in humans and animals.[9] Jaak Panskeep proposed seven basic emotions: seeking, rage, lust, fear, care, panic, and play through observation of animal behavioral responses following electrical stimulation of discrete regions of the brain.[10] In addition to the basic emotions listed by Ekman and Panskeep, there are other emotion categories which have been posited. Significantly, all the lists include the emotion of fear. As more becomes known about emotions, those which are generally accepted will likely be subcategorized and some may be eliminated. In addition to the so-called primary emotions, Damasio has elaborated secondary or social emotions such as embarrassment, jealousy, guilt, and pride.[7]

The acquisition of every biological trait has an evolutionary history. This is, of course, true of emotions and consciousness. A recent book by Joseph LeDoux emphasizes the evolutionary development of defensive and survival circuits from bacteria to humans and makes mention of the fact throughout the book that many of the fundamental mechanisms which have preserved life on earth arose in single-cell microorganisms.[6] Two structures which figure prominently in many theories of emotions and consciousness are the amygdala and the cerebral cortex. An amygdala-like structure with functions and pathways similar to those in mammals is found in fish, reptiles, and birds.[11] In the late 1960s cerebral cortical tissue, though rudimentary, was discovered in even non-vertebrate organisms.[12] Thus, the themes of divergence and diversification may have outflanked the "need" to form entirely novel structures on the path to human complexity.

Proceeding from the defenses bacteria have evolved, another pivotal development on the evolutionary continuum may have begun at the point that organisms were able to sense what Derek Denton and others have called "primordial emotions" deriving from basic survival needs;[13] hunger, thirst, the need to breathe and the sensation of air hunger, core temperature regulation, sensations arising from sexual arousal, pain, the compelling need for sleep after a period of sleeplessness, and other internal biological needs. The sophisticated sensors of these imperatives are part and parcel of development of what Denton terms primary consciousness. He particularly notes the effect that breathing CO_2, stimulating air hunger, has on the attentional systems of the human brain; the imperious, as he calls it, sensation some humans report of panic and even impending death.

The focus on the internal state of the body, and what one is feeling, is called interoception.[14] As we've learned more about interoceptive signals in humans we've gained information about the brain regions which receive these signals. A key area is the insula, though multiple regions receive information about the condition of the body, all in the service of maintaining physiological systems within their functional bounds. The regions inputting these signals may be part of an assembly of widely distributed networks. Concurrently, the internal environment responds in myriad ways to the external milieu. Awareness of the world is probably the most basic level of consciousness. That portion of the external world created by an individual organism, the extended phenotype, is the subject of one of Richard Dawkin's insightful books.[15]

It hardly requires mention that there is no bright line demarcating organisms without consciousness from those deemed to possess this trait. Precursors were present in the animal ancestors from which we evolved, though our knowledge about neural structures and social factors is thin. As will be indicated, not all scholars believe animals have consciousness. Because we don't have a mechanistic definition of consciousness, we speculate and theorize. Embedded within this theory-laden field is the issue of animal capabilities; do any animals have emotions and feelings and have a conscious awareness of these? If any do, how will we know? Of the contemporary investigators previously mentioned, Adolphs, Anderson, Denton, Panskeep, and Damasio hold that some animals are consciously aware of emotions and feelings, though their views are nuanced and must be individually evaluated. An in-depth treatment of their arguments and of others who support similar positions will not be covered herein. LeDoux takes the stance that we do not yet have research findings which would support these assertions, though he is open to the possibility that animals may have consciousness.

The vast literature bearing on this question is a pleasure to read. Many books and articles link animal behavior and consciousness.[16] Popular treatments of the subject are laced with compelling examples reminiscent of animal feeling and emotions.[17] Though I am uncertain on the matter, I am confident research can incrementally get us closer to resolution. I am reminded of the "emotional" outburst/display when our family's pet dog realized (or rather remembered) that crossing the bridge over the Colorado River meant one thing; he was going to the vet. This recall of emotional memory is similar to the recall of both pleasurable and fear memories in mice revealed by optogenetics which was referenced in the last chapter. Detailed behavioral observations, coupled with improving technologies in humans and other species, will aid our quest for answers.

Theory of mind (TOM) has been held out by numerous investigators as one probable indicator of consciousness. TOM is the ability to attribute mental states to oneself and others, states such as intentions, desires, emotions, beliefs, and knowledge. A cardinal feature of TOM is empathy, the capacity to share the affective state of another and to offer consolation. The anterior cingulate cortex (ACC), involved in emotion as well as other higher order cognitive functions, figures prominently in empathy circuits. In great apes, canines, corvids, and elephants, comforting behavior by others of their species has been demonstrated following naturally occurring aggression.

This behavior is also manifest in rodents and can be specified in terms of neural circuits and neurochemistry. Utilizing optogenetics, it was shown that the anterior cingulate cortex (ACC) is a locus of distinct neural pathways which mediate empathy in mice.[18] These investigations involved "demonstrator" mice administered a painful stimulus, followed by relief of the pain, all in the presence of "observer" mice. These observers exhibited an empathic response to both situations. The circuit responsible for these responses in observer mice connected the ACC to the nucleus accumbens, a brain region implicated in the last chapter in reward and depressive states. This study also revealed that a demonstrator mouse subjected to a fear-evoking stimulus would elicit fear reactions in an observer mouse. This latter behavior was the product of a neural circuit from the ACC to the basolateral amygdala, a region implicated in fear generation in multiple studies cited in the last chapter.

Another study was conducted in voles.[19] Prairie voles are socially monogamous rodents, as contrasted with meadow voles, their promiscuous cousins. In contradistinction to meadow voles, if a prairie vole is subjected to Pavlovian fear conditioning, its stressed state will be discerned by its partner, leading to grooming and other comforting behavior. The observer animal mirrors the demonstrator cagemate's stress by also manifesting a fear response and anxiety-related behaviors, as well as elevated corticosterone levels. Additionally, the activity of oxytocin neurons in the ACC was assessed. Oxytocin is known to support affiliative responses in humans. This hormone exerts its actions through its receptor. When a chemical which blocks the oxytocin receptor was infused into the ACC, the empathic responses of observer voles toward partners were eliminated, revealing conservation of empathic behaviors between prairie voles and humans.

These are early days in the attempt to understand emotion. As with other broad swaths of biology, the inclusion of model organisms from the worm (*C. elegans*) and the fruit fly (*Drosophila*), to rodents, mammals, and primates will be utilized. Adolphs and Anderson have proposed that emotions are biological entities they regard as central emotion states. These internal states cause the behavioral, cognitive, and physiological outcomes, not the reverse. They hold that emotion states are distinct from experiences of emotion.[5] Thus, emotions can be studied without interposing that most daunting of traits, consciousness. Though they would contend that feelings are also a consequence of central emotion states and that feelings are subjective experiences of an emotion state reportable only by humans, they reject the notion that this precludes studying emotions in animals. To include other organisms, they have suggested a framework whereby emotions can be investigated from invertebrates to humans.[20] These authors acknowledge Darwin who advanced the intuition that the stridulations produced by insect wings may be an expression of "fear" or "terror," though they concede this is an instance of "unabashed anthropomorphizing."

To avoid the dilemma of imputing labels we associate with human emotion to other organisms, Adolphs and Anderson propose a shift. The focus, they contend, should be on analysis of the underlying neural circuits when observation of behaviors could plausibly have an emotional component. These investigations can be fostered by newer methods for manipulating circuits and recording behavioral readouts.[21] This approach has been successfully employed in the study of mating and aggression in flies and mice, revealing evolutionary links.[22] Though invertebrate circuits may not be homologous to those mediating an emotion in humans, their goal is to discover fundamental properties of "emotional primitives," as they term them, which they propose may have served as evolutionary building blocks of emotion across phylogeny.

As previously mentioned, Adolphs and Anderson join Damasio, Panskeep and others in the belief that animals not only harbor emotions, but that some species have a consciousness of the emotion they are experiencing/feeling. This brings to the fore the question of which brain regions generate emotions? While the study of fear is reasonably advanced, the remaining emotions have not been empirically distinguished. Panskeep, based on his research in which he electrically stimulated certain regions of the brains of animals and elicited responses he interpreted as specific emotions, concluded that emotions emanate from the subcortical region, the collection of nuclei and other structures residing beneath the outer covering of the cerebral cortex with extensive interconnections and tracts to and from various sectors of the cerebral cortex. He identified the loci and neural tracts as "emotion operating systems." He emphasized that the homologies of subcortical structures from species to species, particularly within mammalian groups, are greater than the homology which exists when comparing cerebral cortices. Panskeep also concluded that each of the seven core emotions he elaborated has a dedicated neural circuit through which these emotions manifest.[10] Though the details are disputed, Panskeep, now deceased, remains a respected figure in the field.

Damasio also posits subcortical loci for the generation of emotions. More than others, he has invoked interoception, somewhat in agreement with William James, as a major contributor to emotions. He has proposed neural pathways, based on neuroscience studies, from the brainstem through other relay stations in the subcortex which might plausibly mediate emotions. Emotions, as he averred, are "sandwiched" between the brainstem supporting basic survival functions and the higher cortical regions.[7,23] Damasio and Panskeep believe that emotions are innately expressed from subcortical circuits and have implied that these emotions are intrinsically conscious entities. In Damasio's view, groups of cells are "neurally disposed" to initiate activity resulting in an emotion.

Other investigators invoke the cerebral cortex, arguing that this structure is involved in a fundamental way, particularly in the creation of consciousness through integration of multiple inputs. A severe, fortunately rare human developmental disorder, hydranencephaly, has provided discussion points relevant to emotions and consciousness in humans. It is suspected that hydranencephaly results from the blockage of the major artery, the middle cerebral artery, supplying the developing cortex, usually at some point prior to midgestation, resulting in replacement of nearly all the cortical tissue by fluid. Though each case is distinct, mid-brain structures are largely spared. The children who survive have severe cognitive and motor deficits and parents have often been told that their child will be in a permanent vegetative state.[24]

It has, however, been a revelation to many who have evaluated these children that some survivors exhibit "emotional" behavior, smiling and laughing at appropriate times, responding to the presence of familiar people, and reacting to music and similar stimuli. Some authors have invoked the example of hydranencephaly to argue the cerebral cortex is not necessary for the trait of consciousness.[24, 25] Based on these cases, it might be further argued that the subcortical region is, indeed, the origin of emotion and consciousness without the need for integration in the cerebral cortex. Hydranencephaly can help inform the discussion of the locus of emotion and consciousness, but caution is warranted against overinterpretation of the lessons of this devastating condition which occurs early in gestation, disrupting the links which should have formed. Could the remaining tissue in the mid-brain possibly take on functions not normally performed?

The field of emotion research is fluid. As the science matures, there will be shifts in perspective. A recalibration by LeDoux, long considered one of the most productive and thoughtful scientists evaluating the mechanisms of fear production, the role of the amygdala, and the anxiety which results from prolonged fear, has espoused a notable shift away from the dominant paradigm. He reasons we should eschew a focus on circuits which mediate fear and instead regard them as "defensive or survival circuits."[26] For their part, Adolphs and Anderson have opined that the difference between fear circuits and defense/survival circuits is semantic.[5] LeDoux has, as noted, surveyed the evolutionary history of organisms from bacteria to the development of complex human brains.[6] In his reformulation, the trajectory has not been toward the making of feelings but toward the production of the means to survive. LeDoux (and many others) have repeatedly stressed that single-celled organisms have developed a large suite of defenses to detect and respond to threats. The core of these defenses is the bedrock which has been continuously modified as new challenges have been presented. Of the challenges organisms often confront, evolution has clearly placed a premium on evading predators, a primary driver for the attainment of survival skills. It may be the case that predation on primates and our hominid ancestors was a factor in the development of specialized skills and structures such as language and a large brain.[27] Systems of defense against the possibility of bodily harm and predation are not as necessary today, but unfortunately have left in their evolutionary wake the vigilance mechanisms mediating fear and anxiety.

LeDoux and Lisa Feldman Barrett (see below) provide important, contrasting views of the means by which the brain creates an emotion. There are similarities, but also revealing differences. In both theories, emotions are "built;" cognitively assembled in LeDoux's formulation. In a similar vein, Barrett's model is called the theory of constructed emotion.[28] Though the two systems propose similar elements with which to build emotions, these two investigators differ in the perspectives they take. There are many elements which conceivably serve as building blocks for the creation of an emotion. These include the neural processing of our basic senses conveying information about the external world and signals from our body, activated memory systems, our thoughts and the schema which organize our thoughts, and the representations we have developed of similar past events. Within LeDoux's theory, these elements arise nonconsciously. If a stimulus has produced fear, as an example, this emotion will only be consciously experienced when a self is integrated into the cortical cognitive processes to complete the experience of fear.[3] The necessity of the self for cognitive awareness was emphasized earlier by Damasio.[29] Contemplation of the emotion of fear (or other emotions) is possible in humans, reflected in the capacity for metacognition.

Barrett's theory of constructed emotion posits that the brain utilizes the elements listed above, incorporating the added elements of expectation and prediction of what a developing situation portends. This construction takes place against the background of core affect—valence (pleasantness or unpleasantness) and arousal. However, there are no modules or systems which are innately dedicated to a specific emotion such as fear or anger. In fact, in her system there are no "natural kinds" of emotion.[30] She argues that evolutionarily conserved circuits for basic emotions do not exist. The constructions are assembled for the moment and the situation. Rather than specific emotion modules, the brain has more general processes such as memory, perception, and attention which function in a cultural context to create an emotion. Her socially constructed categories will vary by culture and epoch. Though Barrett does not focus on emotional categories and their neurobiological substrates, her theory has elements of psychology and basic neuroscience, acknowledging the studies which clarify the role of central nervous system structures. Her theory of emotion construction only skirts the realm of consciousness when she describes how emotions are made. Animals, she contends, do not have emotion concepts, which would preclude the utilization of emotion as a component of consciousness. Animals may feel, but do not possess self-awareness of fear in her view.

As the last chapter illustrated, within the domains of learning and memory, anxiety and depression, and now the addition of emotions, familiar regions figure prominently; the amygdala, hippocampus, and the prefrontal cortex. Their functional relationships are clear in the synchronization of brain wave frequencies within these interconnected hubs.[11] In league with cognition, the amygdala participates in emotional learning and memory, involving perception, attention, and social learning.[11, 31] The amygdala is dysregulated by stress and fear, its heightened activity negatively impacting the hippocampus. The hippocampus is also directly vulnerable to stress, particularly impacting its mnemonic functions. Long lasting stress inhibits the production of new neurons (neurogenesis) in the hippocampus, which impairs learning and memory and synaptic plasticity.[32] The prefrontal cortex, the most highly evolved region of the brain, regulates emotions, thoughts, and actions via connections to many other structures. Acute, severe stress impairs these functions of the prefrontal cortex. In this circumstance this region switches from measured, thoughtful regulation to the reflexive and rushed emotional responses of the amygdala and related subcortical structures.[33]

There are a multitude of interconnected brain structures which participate in the functions mentioned in this chapter but have gone unmentioned, many of which participate in stress and fear responses, often via connection with the three major hubs mentioned above. I first became familiar with the anatomic complexity of the brain as a first-year medical student. This appreciation deepened when I helped instruct in the neuroanatomy lab the following year. Neuroanatomy, daunting even as a stand-alone discipline, is the superficial entry into neuroscience. Embedded within the anatomy is complexity on an almost inconceivable scale. The study of stress, fear, anxiety, depression, and emotion bring a portion of this complexity into stark relief as more research results are amassed.

Whereas many emotion researchers have invoked consciousness when discussing emotion, LeDoux has been expansive on this matter. Whether there will ever be a scientifically credible explanation for consciousness, LeDoux has been willing to join others in at least laying the groundwork for this endeavor. His history of research on fear mechanisms has led to his modifications of a theory of consciousness called HOT (higher order theory).[34] He utilizes the emotion of fear to illustrate his formulation of the theory.[35] Fear learning is an instructive model to utilize. It sheds light on interactions between emotional and cognitive processes in the brain. Additionally, all fears, including fears born of imagination or introspection (existential fears), use similar neural systems.[36] The underlying perspectives in LeDoux's theory run counter to the notion that emotions are innately generated and experienced via subcortical circuits. In this theory, emotions are not intrinsically conscious at that level. Rather, representations of a threat are instantiated in higher order circuits after activation of relevant long-term memories and one's personal emotion schema produce lower order, nonconscious representations. When cortical (higher order) circuits process these lower order representations, the emotion of fear is consciously experienced in humans.

In the higher order theory there is a single, general cortical system that produces conscious experiences. Emotion does not occupy a privileged position. An emotion is processed like any conscious experience such as a visual scene. The higher order processing of the myriad inputs from other brain regions destined to enter the steam of consciousness is orchestrated primarily by subregions of the prefrontal cortex. The means of producing consciousness incorporates cognitive processes such as attention and working memory so the representations can be retained and thought about (metacognition). All of this is underpinned by a representation of self. In

LeDoux's view, animals cannot be said, at least at this time, to have conscious awareness because of the inability to hold in mind and to verbalize self-referential material. Although animals may demonstrate outward manifestations which resemble emotional behavior in humans, LeDoux argues that unless or until science can demonstrate that these behaviors reflect states of consciousness, nonconscious interpretations would be the prudent, default stance.

⁞⁞⁞

I HAVE frequently referenced the writing of LeDoux because he has, for many decades, established a theme I had been contemplating prior to reading this author. He has forged a chain which begins with fear as a core emotion that ultimately links to consciousness.[37] He has written that this is a process of "creeping up on consciousness".[6] I have borrowed from this perspective in the chapter's title. There has been, along this evolutionary path, an inestimable number of "innovations"/variations which have given the possessors both grief and advantages, the entire gamut hastening the emergence of consciousness.

It is my purpose in the latter part of this chapter to attempt a further exploration of this link, drawing upon the field of stem cell research. I will begin this discussion with the topic of neurogenesis, the creation of new neurons in the brain. Neurogenesis ties to subjects which have already been stressed, including learning and memory. After explicating the association between neurogenesis and depression, I will extend the subject to include brain "organoids," a recapitulation in the laboratory of portions of the brain reminiscent of embryological brain development, starting with either embryonic stem cells or induced pluripotent stem cells (iPSCs) mentioned in the personal narrative. For this concluding portion of the chapter, I beseech your indulgence as I depart from scientific rigor by suggesting an inquiry—likely one far in the future—into brain organoid research and fear, a possible wedge into the intricacies of consciousness.

Neurogenesis bespeaks the plasticity of the brain. It was not widely accepted that neurogenesis occurs until the 1990s, though evidence for its existence was published as early as 1965.[38] Stem cells are known to populate organs throughout the body to serve as a source for tissue maintenance and repair. These progenitors, through the multi-step process of maturation, are the cells which produce, for instance, the multitude of blood cells following differentiation. Differentiation or maturation of stem cells is reliant upon the local environment, the niche, as well as multiple other factors to specify distinct, fully differentiated cell types, a process termed fate determination.

Until recently, as mentioned, it had been thought that the brain was static in the sense that no new cells contributed to the staggering functions of this organ. By this reasoning, all neurons were derived during embryologic development. Newer methods have, however, clearly documented that neurogenesis occurs in two regions of the rodent brain, one region contributing new neurons to olfaction, the other contributing these cells to the dentate gyrus in the hippocampus. Neurogenesis has also been documented in the hippocampus of humans by an imaginative study which took advantage of dating techniques used in archeology.[39] The research is based on the significant increase in global levels of Carbon-14 that resulted from the above-ground testing of nuclear weapons during the Cold War in the 1950s and 1960s, declining after 1963 following a ban on such testing. The Carbon-14 was taken up by plants via CO_2 during photosynthesis and made its way into humans who ate the plants or animals grazing on the plants. The Carbon-14 was incorporated into newly synthesized DNA during cell division in trace amounts, proportional to environmental levels. Thus, assessment of these levels could be a "time stamp" for the birth of a cell. For this research, the brains of deceased individuals willed for the purpose of assessing the Carbon-14 levels in neurons in the hippocampus were studied. The studies proved that neurogenesis occurs in the adult brain throughout life. The process of adding new, plastic neurons which become incorporated into the existing circuitry of the hippocampus has proven to be of marked importance for mood and cognition, as discussed below.

New neurons lend a dynamism to the central nervous system. Their role in memory formation is central to this dynamism. Fred Gage has been on the front lines of neurogenesis research, contributing basic science insights and thoughtful reviews concerning the manner by which new neurons are regulated as these cells participate in learning and mood.[40] The generation and function of these cells involves a complex host of interacting factors, including crosstalk among morphogens (signaling molecules that direct tissue development), neuromodulators such as serotonin, neurotropic factors such as BDNF, neurotransmitters such as glutamate, and hormones such as the glucocorticoids.[41, 42] A specialized niche in which the stem cells reside also contributes nutritive elements. Other key regulators include electrical transmission or activity,[43] and changes in the epigenetic landscape as stem cells go from a naïve state to a fully differentiated state, leading ultimately to incorporation into the existing hippocampal circuitry.[44] Entering and exiting connections to and from the hippocampus to the amygdala, prefrontal cortex, and other brain regions will be established by the new neurons for learning and mood regulation, along with the intrahippocampal connections these neurons establish.

Many of the studies on the beneficial effects of neurogenesis utilize rodents as subjects. The extent of neurogenesis can be specified in these species by incorporating bromodeoxyuridine (BrdU), an analogue of thymidine, into DNA, thereby tagging cells undergoing mitosis, including neural stem cells and their progeny. Levels of adult neurogenesis are increased by measures which enhance learning,[45] assessed by tests previously discussed. Neurogenesis is also increased by environmental richness and exercise.[46] The environmentally enriched cage is larger, housing more animals for social engagement, has tunnels and novel objects to explore, and has a running wheel for exercise. Mice voluntarily spend hours a day on the running wheel, which alone increases neurogenesis and learning, even in aged mice.[47]

The case has been made that these interventions increase neurogenesis and learning. However, it had been unknown whether an intervention which selectively increased neurogenesis was sufficient to increase cognition and improve mood. To address this question, neurogenesis was increased in mice by means of genetic manipulation.[48] On most measures of learning, including spatial learning and contextual fear conditioning, the mice with increased neurogenesis performed like normal controls. However, on one measure, differentiating between overlapping contextual representations, these mice performed better. Thus, their performance improved when discriminating between similar contexts, a process called pattern separation. Pattern separation is implicated in learning and affective disorders, most prominently anxiety.

As has been extensively detailed, the hippocampus is central to memory formation. Investigations are ongoing to determine the function of new neurons in creating memories. In one study a method was utilized which destroyed newly created neurons in mice after a memory trace had been established.[49] The memory involved finding a submerged platform. The location, representing safety, was cued by a visual pattern on the wall of the water tank, as noted in the last chapter. After the training sessions in which the mice learned the pattern which led them to the platform, a toxin was injected which killed the recently generated neurons. In subsequent trials, the mice could remember that a hidden platform was near a patterned visual display—just not which one of the many patterns displayed on the walls. The authors concluded that new neurons form a "critical and enduring component of memories," essential to prevent degradation and to preserve the finer details of memory.

Imaging studies in the 1990s revealed that hippocampal volumes are lower in depressed patient,[50] though it is unclear whether the decrease in neurogenesis consequent to depression could account for this finding. Gage, along with his colleagues, brought increased attention to the association between adult brain neurogenesis and depression in 2000,[51] an association which has been strengthened over succeeding years. It was first shown that chronic treatment of rats with different classes of antidepressants, including those affecting serotonin and norepinephrine actions, and administration of electroconvulsive seizures, increased neurogenesis.[52] Administration of a psychotropic drug without antidepressant activity did not increase neurogenesis. It required chronic treatment, 14 or 28 days, to increase neurogenesis, a time frame which correlates with the delay required for a therapeutic effect of antidepressants.

In addition to the method previously cited to decrease neurogenesis,[49] X-irradiation delivered to the region of the hippocampus which generates new neurons is another method to halt neurogenesis. This method was utilized to evaluate a behavior in mice based on an animal's reluctance to retrieve food pellets from brightly lit areas. This hesitancy is responsive to antidepressants. If neurogenesis is thwarted by X-irradiation, the reluctance to feed is restored despite antidepressants.[53]

The relationship between neurogenesis and depression is compelling, as is the knowledge that the common inciting event(s) for depression is stress. There are multiple ways to apply stress in rodents and hence model depression. These include methods previously discussed: unpredictable mild stress, chronic corticosterone treatment, the social defeat paradigm wherein a mouse is introduced into the territory of a mouse from a larger, more aggressive strain, and others. These and multiple other factors inform the research yet to be accomplished.[54] In humans the common inciting event(s) is also stress, often self-selected or imposed,[55] which must surely deepen the distress.

From the foregoing, an important question arises; can it be determined if neurogenesis buffers stress responses, thereby ameliorating depressive behavior? A key feature predisposing to depression is activation of the main stress pathway, the hypothalamus to pituitary to adrenal gland where glucocorticoids are secreted (cortisone in humans, corticosterone in rodents). When a stress response is triggered, the hippocampus sends a shut-off signal to the hypothalamus when the stressing event (danger) has passed. This regulation requires the production of new neurons.[56] When methods are employed to halt the generation of new neurons, glucocorticoid levels remain elevated for a longer period after bouts of stress induced by restraint. Therefore, the feedback loop is dysregulated. Other tests previously discussed, including the forced swim test which can indicate behavioral despair, decreased preference for sucrose suggesting anhedonia, and decreased food intake in a novel environment are all dysregulated when neurogenesis is impaired, suggesting a depressive state. These studies reveal that neurogenesis buffers stress responses. It is worth noting again that dysregulation of glucocorticoid release is associated not only with depression, but also with cognitive deficits.[57]

Hippocampal anatomy is also a factor. This region consists of a dorsal or superior sector which is more involved with cognition and memory of spatial features, whereas the inferior ventral region is implicated in mood regulation. Thus, it is significant that a group of cells were identified in the ventral hippocampus which were found to be the mediators of stress resilience owing to neurogenesis.[58] The authors speculated that variability in the activity of the hippocampus, specifically cells in the dentate gyrus, could be a major factor determining vulnerability and/or resilience to stress.

Studies on the relative contributions of genetics versus environment to traits such as personality and disease often rely upon twins, dizygotic (fraternal twins) and monozygotic (identical twins) raised together or apart. A revealing murine study could be a model to tease out the variable biological contributions to stress vulnerability. Forty mice from an inbred strain, and therefore genetically identical, were collectively raised in a large, enriched environment. Over the course of three months the mice diverged significantly in exploratory activity, signifying differences in brain plasticity and accompanying behavior between the diverging groups of mice. This difference correlated with the extent of neurogenesis; the greater the production of new neurons the greater the extent of brain plasticity and exploration of their environment.[59]

❖❖❖

EMBRYOLOGY, the unfolding of the developmental program resulting in a fully formed organism, is a wonder of enduring fascination. An understanding of the mechanisms of development has been a major impetus to study differentiation *in vitro*. Studies on specific cell types differentiated in the laboratory have proliferated. The ability to form portions of organs, called "organoids," displaying the structure and function of intact organs has accelerated progress in the stem cell field. This has allowed the investigation of diseases in humans at a more granular level than would otherwise be possible. This aspect and other possibilities of stem cell/organoid research will be offered in the following section.

The foundational principle which allows stem cells to build organisms is self-organization. Examples are everywhere in nature. In 1907 Wilson demonstrated that the cells of a sponge, when completely disaggregated, spontaneously reaggregate to form an intact sponge.[60] In species closer to humans, we distinguish between embryonic stem cells which are pluripotent and can give rise to any cell in the body and adult stem cells which are restricted to specific tissues where they can regenerate that specific tissue when damaged, but not other tissues. Planaria, a tiny flatworm, represents the development of another interesting regenerative cell, the neoblast. Some species of planaria maintain a supply of these stem cells which can regenerate the complete organism from severed pieces. It has been shown that neoblasts blur the boundary between embryonic and adult stem cells. These cells are pluripotent, but nonetheless function as adult stem cells.[61] The stem cells underlying self-organization are a malleable, diverse lot.

This tissue-forming disposition of stem cells, as previously noted, was first displayed to me when Dr. Maeda urged that I look at an embryoid body, a group of cells that form in a tissue culture dish of mouse embryonic stem cells (mESCs). Embryoid bodies also form when human embryonic stem cells (hESCs) are cultured. Peering down the microscope it was evident that in one embryoid body a portion of the tissue had spontaneously organized cardiac muscle cells which had electrically coupled and begun to rhythmically contract. When a previously homogeneous group of cells within an embryoid body converts to a different state, this is called symmetry breaking, a key concept in many branches of science, including physics.

One clear way to determine that ES cells are pluripotent is to implant a small cluster under the skin of a mouse. Pluripotent cells will form a nonmalignant tumor called a teratoma which has derivatives of the three germ layers, endoderm, ectoderm, and mesoderm such as teeth, hair, brain, muscle, bone, and others. Teratomas can also form from primordial germ cells within an ovary. I have been at the surgeries of several of these unusual cases. An intrinsic developmental program is randomly initiated in a cell or group of cells, leading to multiple compartments within the tumor containing a single, self-organized tissue without external instructions. Teratomas can also occur in other parts of the body and may first present during the fetal period on ultrasound, most commonly a growth protruding from the lower portion of the fetal spine called a sacrococcygeal teratoma.

Protocols have been developed to differentiate murine induced pluripotent (miPSCs) and human induced pluripotent stem cells (hiPSCs), along with mESCs and hESCs, into specific cell types in a tissue culture dish. These differentiation protocols have relied upon experimentation and knowledge of embryology. They require a supportive media, applying a cocktail of chemicals, including growth factors and others, at the right time and amount to nudge the cells in a chosen direction. Though a multitude of cell types can be derived, I will concentrate on differentiation of neurons from pluripotent cells and the potential to learn from these cells. To derive neurons (or any other cell type), investigators try to simulate *in vivo* neurogenesis to the extent possible. Fortunately for neuroscientists interested in this field, neurons are among the cell types which are relatively easy to derive. The ability to generate human neurons has already contributed to a deeper knowledge of psychiatric diseases.[62] The following examples illustrate the range of studies and principal findings on common psychiatric disorders. Recall that when hiPSCs are utilized, the neurons in the dish are derived from individual patients.

Gage and his group reported the first study of patients with schizophrenia, a highly heritable disorder characterized by hallucinations, delusions, and cognitive defects. Using iPSCs, they surveyed the proteins expressed at the synapses, the growth of axons, dendrites, and the density of synapses, neural transmission characteristics, and gene expression profiles of these neurons.[63] Basic electrophysiology was normal, though the connections these neurons established were diminished. There was a reduction in the levels of synaptic proteins, possibly reflecting a decrease in synaptic density. Gene analysis revealed altered expression of many proteins within key signaling pathways. The deficits in neuronal connectivity were reversed following treatment of these neurons with the antipsychotic medication loxapine.

Schizophrenia, like Parkinson disease and many others, is associated with multiple genetic alterations. Different combinations of genes, interacting with environmental influences, predispose to the illness. However, Parkinson disease and schizophrenia can uncommonly be attributed to mutations in a single gene. Rare families in which a mutation in the DISC1 gene (disrupted in schizophrenia 1) is present have been studied by means of iPSC technology.[64] The results support other studies which found that there was decreased synaptic connectivity in forebrain neurons and altered regulation of many genes related to synaptic function. Neurotransmitters are released from vesicles in the presynaptic region of the neuron. In the face of a mutant DISC1 protein, release was defective. The results, including the finding that genes important for synaptic function are dysregulated, lend weight to the theory that schizophrenia is a "disease of synapses."[65]

Induced PSCs have also assisted in understanding bipolar disorder.[66] Individuals with this psychiatric disease experience bouts of depression which alternate with periods of mania. Some, but not all, patients respond favorably to lithium. Fibroblasts were dedifferentiated to iPSCs from patients with bipolar disorder and from healthy controls. These iPSCs were subsequently converted to neurons resembling a population of hippocampal neurons. There was an increase of neuronal activity, a hyperexcitability measured by action potential firing. It may be significant that mitochondrial function, assayed by gene expression studies, was augmented. Enhanced mitochondrial function will supply more energy for neuronal firing. The studies were performed on both lithium responders and lithium non-responders. The electrophysiologic and mitochondrial changes were normalized when lithium was added, but only in the neurons of lithium responders, adding validity to the findings.

Advancements in stem cell research have been fueled by the increasing ability to convert stem cells into a pure population of fully differentiated cell types, both for basic investigations and potential therapies. Mention has been made of the differentiation of hiPSCs into neurons which function in the dopamine pathways and the therapeutic effect these dopaminergic neurons showed when injected into the brains of a primate model of Parkinson disease.[67] Neurons functioning in serotonin pathways (serotonergic neurons) have also been generated, providing the cellular material to study depression. Serotonergic neurotransmission is altered in depression and selective serotonin reuptake inhibitors (SSRIs) are prescribed. These drugs delay the reentry of serotonin from the synaptic cleft into neurons, thus prolonging its action.

Unfortunately, SSRIs do not work in many depressed patients. The Gage group studied serotonergic neurons derived from iPSCs of SSRI responders and non-responders.[68] Out of hundreds of patients with major depressive disorder available for this study, the investigators chose to interrogate the serotonergic neurons of three patients responding well to an SSRI compared to the neurons of three non-responders. The neurons from this latter group displayed a relationship between a protocadherin gene cluster and aberrant structure of serotonergic neurons, including neurite (axon and dendrite) growth. To lend credence to the findings, when the function of this protocadherin gene cluster is decreased in serotonergic neurons by genetic manipulation in intact mice, these neurons become disorganized, and the brain is inappropriately wired by the serotonergic circuits which travel widely in the brain. If the gene cluster is completely inactivated in serotonergic neurons in mice, the altered circuitry is associated with depressive behaviors.[69] The complementarity of genetic studies in living mice and human tissue culture studies is well illustrated by these studies. The ability to obtain a specific cell type, such as a population of serotonergic neurons, from pluripotent stem cells has provided the opportunity to model diseases closer to the source and the potential to supply cells which may be of therapeutic benefit if delivered to a diseased organ.

⁂

THE BASIC science and therapeutic possibilities of stem cell research have been significantly advanced with the development of organoids. These structures, as indicated, are miniature replicas which recapitulate aspects of the structure and function of the intact organ. Organoids are cultured in a three-dimensional (3D) environment which provides a greater opportunity for cells and groups of cells to express the intrinsic capacity to respond to mechanical and chemical cues—some of these imposed by the investigators—to create physiologically relevant tissues. Culturing on a flat, plastic dish (2D) does not permit the same degree of developmental complexity. Beginning with a population of stem cells of murine or human origin, these cells are directed along pathways which mimic, to the extent possible, the embryological development of the specified organ. Though it is early days for this field, the extant results from the marriage of tissue engineering principles[70, 71] and stem cell biology promise a future of continuing discovery. There is understandable enthusiasm for the potential to use this technology to develop new drugs and perform the requisite safely studies. This can be expanded to personalized medicine, the capacity to grow iPSC lines to test the efficacy of a drug in the tissues of an affected individual, or to derive cells or even organoids for transplantation without the concern for immune rejection when iPSCs are cultured. This technology is also lessening the need for animal experimentation.

Successfully growing organoids has relied upon the science of embryology to simulate the relevant developmental steps and processes. This requires knowledge of the signaling pathways, when to inhibit and when to activate and with what mix of morphogens and growth factors, and during what temporal window. Development often requires morphogen gradients, higher to lower concentrations to pattern the tissues. There are methods to establish gradients, though organoids may do so intrinsically. The knowledge to target the robust regulatory systems directing development toward organoid formation has been incrementally obtained.[72] Hydrogels and scaffolds of a variety of biomaterials have been utilized. Vascularizing the tissues in culture is an ongoing effort.[73] Mechanical forces play a large role, particularly those in the extracellular matrix mediated by mesenchymal cells.[74]

A Japanese group combined many of these elements to create human organ buds representing pancreas, kidney, intestine, heart, lung, and brain, utilizing diverse cell types and mesenchymal cells to condense the initial cell population and begin the process of organ bud formation.[75] The buds, containing cells which form blood vessels, were subsequently vascularized by transplantation into immunodeficient mice, thus preventing rejection. Future possibilities include vascularization of these structures in animals such as the pig, allowing growth of larger organoids for transplantation. Many hurdles, however, remain.

In addition to the generation of tissue buds, ongoing research has provided the means to develop 3D organoids representing many human tissues.[76] Much work has focused on intestinal organoids. It is noteworthy that a single intestinal stem cell, present in the tissue for reparative purposes, can produce a 3D intestinal organoid,[77] attesting to the regenerative power of even adult stem cells. In addition to the importance of developing methods to vascularize organoids in culture, a nerve supply is also important, particularly for gastrointestinal applications. By combining hESC-derived neural crest cells with developing intestinal tissues, a nervous system was established which led to coordinated wave-like propagations.[78]

Intestinal tissue supplied the first example of organoid development in the service of personalized medicine.[79] Cystic fibrosis (CF) has protean manifestations, including adverse gastrointestinal effects. The disorder is caused by over a thousand different mutations in a single gene encoding a channel that transports chloride. Mucus secretions become thick and viscous when the channel is defective, leading to respiratory and other problems. Intestinal organoids with a defective chloride channel from a patient with a rare CF mutation were grown from iPSCs. Drugs with a therapeutic effect in other patients with CF were screened for efficacy in this organoid model. The channel proved responsive to one of these drugs.

Many luminaries have contributed to stem cell research. Yoshiki Sasai will be remembered for first proposing that pluripotent stem cells could generate organized and highly complex 3D tissues resembling their *in vivo* counterparts. This visionary ideal has been particularly successful for the generation of brain organoids.[80] Sasai's contributions to brain organoid formation have been pioneering. His group first generated forebrain structures, followed shortly by specific brain regions such as a six-layered neocortex, cerebellum, hippocampus, anterior pituitary gland, and other defined brain regions.[81] The anterior pituitary gland his group generated was functional, responding to releasing factors from the hypothalamus and secreting ACTH which stimulated corticosterone secretion from the adrenal gland. When this tissue was grafted into mice with hypopituitarism, the grafts responded to the appropriate signals, prolonging the lives of these mice.[82]

Sasai and his group also promulgated the principles which govern the *in vitro* levels of complexity they achieved.[83] His contributions to the field center on self-organization, a principle of development dependent upon the intrinsic capacity of cells to sense and respond to mechanical forces and chemical cues such as morphogen gradients. These innate qualities are evocative of those displayed by bacteria, discussed in the chapter Microbes under topics such as quorum sensing. Sasai defined three sequential modes of tissue self-organization; self-assembly, or the control of relative cell positions by local rules of development; self-patterning, or the spontaneous organization of complex tissue patterns without external cues; and self-driven morphogenesis, or the formation of complex tissue shapes driven by intrinsic mechanisms. Many specific brain regions have been formed via these three fundamental processes.

Organoid formation could serve as a model to study the complexity that is demonstrated in biological and non-biological systems. Underpinning this complexity is self-organization, as mentioned, a feature rife in the biological sciences.[84] A related theme, emergence, the concept that the whole is more complex than the sum of its interacting parts, is another feature of inestimable significance for the stem cell field. Indeed, Sasai has proposed the term "emergence biology" for this research field.[83] Emergence has a deep history in the annals of biological thought.[85] Emergence biology adds a rich layer to the basic concept of emergence.

Advances and refinements in organoid technology are proceeding. Organ-on-a-chip is a microfluidic cell culture device with perfused chambers in which tissue-level and organ-level physiology are displayed following assembly on a synthetic matrix.[86] This technology furthers the prospect of probing tissue interactions. Some organoids are cultured in spinning bioreactors which improve nutrient and oxygen exchange. Producing consistency in organoid structure and function from cell line to cell line and experiment to experiment has been an issue. Modeling human brain disorders would be problematic unless there was consistency across different cell lines and procedures. Improvements have been realized. For example, utilizing single cell RNA sequencing from organoids representing different cell lines and regions of the cerebral cortex, one group showed that the diversity of cell types within organoids reliably reproduced the cellular diversity of the developing human cerebral cortex.[87]

As the field has advanced, brain organoids have proven valuable in understanding some aspects of enigmatic disorders such as autism and microcephaly (small brain). Autism is a disorder of brain development, thought to begin in the fetal period. Etiological factors have been identified, but about 80 percent of cases have no known cause. In one revelatory study, iPSC lines were derived from patients with autism with no clear etiology. Brain organoids from these lines representing fetal telencephalon (which forms the cerebrum) from around midgestation were generated. The major finding was an increased production of inhibitory neurons which use gamma-aminobutyric acid (GABA) as neurotransmitter. The mechanism of this overproduction was attributed to an increased expression of the FOXG1 gene.[88]

Another disorder which occurs during fetal brain development is microcephaly, a brain much smaller than normal, associated with significant developmental disability. There are single gene causes as well as idiopathic cases (of unknown cause). To effectively study microcephaly, one group of scientists first optimized cerebral organoids, utilizing hESCs, spinning bioreactors, and growth in Matrigel. These organoids developed discrete, interdependent regional identities. Organization of the cortex replicated that in humans. They then studied a patient with microcephaly due to a single gene mutation.[89] The main finding in these iPSC-derived organoids was premature neuronal differentiation in the progenitor zones of the developing cerebral cortex. It was surmised that these founding populations of neurons, the progenitors, do not expand to the extent they do in normally developing brains, leading to smaller structures. Another category of causes for microcephaly is, rarely, a maternal viral infection which crosses the placenta to infect the fetus. A relatively recent example with adverse consequences is the Zika virus. Investigators first optimized iPSC organoid formation in bioreactors. They then exposed developing brain organoids to the Zika virus. As a result, one of the neurogenic zones, the ventricular zone of the cerebral cortex, was shown to be markedly reduced, likely as a result of cell death and suppression of neural progenitor cell proliferation.[90]

The importance of genetic and environmental factors in disease causation has been emphasized. To minimize the effect of these factors, the study of identical twins raised together is optimal. A group studied forebrain neurons from iPSC-derived organoids of identical twins discordant for psychosis. Their single-cell analyses revealed several findings of note.[91] RNA sequencing, the method to determine the proteins manufactured by a cell, showed increased GABA specification. GABA is an inhibitory neurotransmitter. Thus, there existed an excitation-inhibition imbalance. There was also decreased cell proliferation associated with diminished signaling in a key developmental pathway.

Multiple studies, some cited above, have demonstrated that specific regions of the brain can be generated. This has led to another technological step toward greater complexity in organoid research, the fusion of brain regions to study the extent to which these "assembloids" integrate in a functionally realistic way. In one study the dorsal or superior forebrain region was fused with the ventral or inferior region. Functional neurons from the ventral region, called interneurons, migrated into the dorsal region as occurs during fetal brain development. Inhibitory and excitatory neural activity was documented.[92] This system was used to study Timothy syndrome, a single gene disorder affecting many organ systems, including prominent neurological and developmental defects. The scientists found that the migration of interneurons from the ventral to dorsal region was defective.

Can the fusion of brain regions provide information on disorders as complex as depression? The thalamus functions as a relay station, connecting peripheral sense organs to areas of the cortex and other regions. Recall that when rodents are fear conditioned a loud sound, the conditioned stimulus, is sent from the thalamus to the dorsolateral amygdala. The thalamus plays a role in major depressive disorder. An MRI study revealed abnormal (increased) connectivity between the medial thalamus and the somatosensory cortex and the temporal lobe in depressed patients. The increase was most prominent between thalamus and the temporal region, with a greater increase as the severity of depression increased.[93] It is significant that the temporal region houses the amygdala and hippocampus.

Thalamic organoids can be generated. These organoids with thalamic architecture and cellular composition can be fused with cerebral organoids. These fused organoids establish functional, reciprocal neural connections.

We know that the origin of any complex developmental disorder or psychiatric disease is not localized to a specific region of the brain. Knowledge of a disease like depression will deepen as more neurochemical circuits are able to cross communicate. A thalamic organoid fused with a cerebral organoid is an initial model with the potential to impact depression research.[94]

Another compelling use of stem cells has been validated. These cells can serve as a vehicle for genetic engineering purposes.[95] At the most basic level a gene mutation can be introduced, or a mutated gene corrected, by the CRISPR/Cas9 complex. This was done for cystic fibrosis, correcting the mutant version of the gene in the stem cells which were then utilized to form an intestinal organoid.[96] This example is one of many illustrating that gene-corrected stem cells and transplantation could one day offer promise for some patients.

An additional creative combination of stem cell and CRISPR/Cas9 technologies has arisen. GWAS (genome-wide association studies) are offering a myriad of genetic variants which are not, acting alone, causative of a particular disease but can contribute to causation. For many disorders multiple genetic variants, acting in concert, are causative. To attempt to determine the effect of a variant on a specific tissue, this variant can be engineered into an iPSC line(s). Gene-edited stem cell lines and unaltered lines from the same individual, along with the resulting differentiated cells and organoids, can then be studied. Since there is considerable background variation in the DNA sequence from one individual to another, this approach is more rigorous when altered and unaltered organoids from the same individual are evaluated. This provides another measure of validity.

Genetic variation and its manipulation can also contribute to our fascination with extinct hominids, principally Neanderthals and Denisovans with which we share a small fraction of our genomes due to interbreeding tens of thousands of years ago. This interest has only grown since the genomes of these two lineages were sequenced to near-completeness. This has allowed a search of data bases for genes expressed in the brain which may have had relevance for complex brain development in modern humans. Based on numerous considerations, one group of investigators selected a variant of the NOVA1 gene. The DNA version found in Denisovans and Neanderthals contains a single nucleotide difference from the human version, changing one amino acid in the encoded protein. Genome-editing was readily accomplished in hESCs. Organoids representing the cortex were grown for several months. The results of this single amino acid change were striking.[97] The "Neanderthal" and "Denisovan" organoids were smaller and had "bumpy" surfaces compared with the smooth surfaces of human organoids at this *in vivo* stage of development. The neurons of the "archaic" organoids migrated more rapidly and their firings were less orderly. Several hundred genes known to affect neuronal development and connectivity showed altered expression. This study previews what will doubtless be a flurry of attempts to chart the genetic pathways that eventuated in the complexity of human thought.

⁝⁝⁝

I AM interested in the possibility of linking the themes of these chapters to brain organoid research and, beyond that, to extend the results of this linkage to any insights into consciousness which may be gained. In the preceding section I attempted to provide sufficient detail on brain organoids to reveal their complexity and thereby to provide these stated goals with a measure of plausibility. In that spirit, the remainder of the chapter is offered in a futuristic, aspirational manner.

First, however, another highly personal detour will assist this effort. When I experienced panic attacks as one manifestation of anxiety and depression, this state of fear was troubling in the extreme. Adjectives can be appended to an episode of panic, but no word or phrase would be sufficient. It is called a panic "attack," an apt term that I will use. A full-blown panic attack abruptly shifts the mental state in a manner analogous to a phase transition—boiling water becoming steam is a readily visualized example wherein one physical state transitions into another physical state. A panic attack may validly represent a phase transition. The experience is not, of course, limited to the brain. Agitation, a racing heart, and other bodily manifestations accompany panic. A person experiencing panic attacks will go to great lengths to avoid the dread which may herald another episode.

These attacks are short-lived, but for that duration, as several commentators have noted, the brain is seized; rational thought is subverted, consciousness is shredded, all mental effort is devoted to the reestablishment of the state that existed prior to this invasion. This fevered effort has the goal of achieving homeostasis, a term coined by Walter Cannon.[98] Homeostasis is realized when the altered physiology is again stable. When order was restored after the first episode I experienced in medical school, I was left with the foreboding that existence had taken a frightful turn. At least this was my sense. I had not had a panic attack since the episode in high school, one provoked while mummified in a rolled-up mat. However, as I also related in the personal narrative, there was a perception of profound mystery and curiosity. What just happened? What jumbled neurochemistry, altered neurotransmission, disordered brain rhythms must have accompanied this malignant occupancy? Perhaps I overdramatize, but many decades later the memories are strong, and these questions persist.

Scientists have a lot to learn about panic. It is sensible to think that MRI could reveal much about a panic attack, at least the anatomic loci on which to focus attention. But episodes are too unpredictable to capture by MRI, and if one had a panic attack due to claustrophobia in an MRI machine, the accompanying movement would degrade the images. The work of Derek Denton was introduced in the beginning portion of this chapter, including the theory that primal emotions such as air hunger, triggered by basic survival systems, were among the elements constituting the primitive origin of consciousness. It is known that breathing a mixture which contains elevated levels of CO_2 precipitates air hunger and, additionally, panicky feelings and outright panic in susceptible people. Denton's group utilized PET (positron emission tomography) scanning in healthy subjects breathing elevated levels of CO_2. The results were predicated on changes in blood flow patterns. In those with panic or panicky symptoms, increased activity was seen widely in subcortical regions, with decreased activity in the executive, "thinking" regions, including the prefrontal cortex and portions of the cingulate cortex.[99] This suggests that a study of panic disorder could not focus on a single region of the brain such as the amygdala.

Additional information questioning a known, specific locus for panic comes from studying patient S.M. whose history is well known in the neuroscience community. She has bilateral amygdala damage, as previously referenced, and, as a consequence, does not evince behavioral or verbal evidence that she experiences the emotion of fear. She can define the emotion and recognizes the behavioral responses of others experiencing fear. However, when she is shown snakes, spiders, horror movies, and other external threats which evoke fear in others, she does not display this emotion. She reportedly had no fear when robbed at knife point. However, when she was challenged with an internal threat, breathing an elevated level of CO_2, she developed air hunger, gasped for air, and attempted to escape by ripping off her breathing mask. She described the experience as very distressing (as "panic") and novel for her. Two other patients, identical twin sisters with amygdala damage, had the same reactions when breathing a mixture containing higher CO_2 concentrations.[100] The sense that they were suffocating produced an intense reaction. The authors suggest that internal threats may be processed in humans differently than threats from the outside.

Investigators at the University of Iowa have been at the forefront of research which has shown a link between the acid-base status of the brain and panic disorder. CO_2, among other agents, is a means to acidify the extracellular environment, providing a route to uncover panic-inducing mechanisms.[101] These colleagues have studied ASIC1a, a gene previously cited in Chapter 1 which is highly expressed in the murine fear circuit. ASIC1a is an acid-sensing ion channel responsible for acid-evoked neural transmission. The channel is "gated"—opened or closed—by proton receptors.[102] Thus, that most fundamental of particles, the proton, is primarily responsible for the function of ASIC1a. Protons (equivalent to positively charged hydrogen ions) also modulate the activity of other receptors in the brain.

Research in mice reveals that the amygdala directly detects CO_2 and acidosis to produce fear behaviors in this species.[103] Following this study which showed the amygdala "senses" acidic changes to elicit defensive reactions, ASIC1a became a focus of increased attention.[104] As noted in the personal narrative, LeDoux cited acid-sensing channels in his book *Anxious* as an emerging area of interest in the quest to understand anxiety.

When the gene coding for the ASIC1a channel was inactivated in mice by the methods revealed in the personal narrative, these mice displayed reduced innate fear, spending more time in the center of an open area and freezing less to a foot shock. They also responded less to a predator odor.[105] When genetic manipulation increased the expression of ASIC1a, fear-related behavior in these mice also increased.[106] Thus, this channel may be important in conferring resilience or predisposition to fear and anxiety. Depression is also affected by ASIC1a function. Inactivating ASIC1a or inhibiting this channel pharmacologically produced antidepressant effects, utilizing the appropriate tests which have been described previously. Restoring lost ASIC1a activity in the amygdala by injecting a virus carrying the gene into this region reversed the antidepressant actions.[107]

When this channel was inactivated there was, additionally, an adverse effect on learning and memory and on the marker for these cognitive functions, synaptic plasticity, demonstrated by impaired long-term potentiation (LTP). These mice also showed spatial learning deficits in the sunken platform test.[108] A finding of note is the effect of ASIC1a on the density of dendrites in hippocampal neurons. Dendrites are knobby projections which receive input from neuronal axons and participate in learning and memory. Decreased ASIC1a decreases dendrite numbers, whereas an increase in the protein increases dendrite numbers.[109]

ASIC1a is as an example of a single protein among many which functions in the domains of learning, memory, emotion, and affective disorders. The investigators who have been working on ASIC1a also posit that changes in acid-base status, even rapidly occurring changes, could be another significant signaling mechanism in the brain. When the assertion is made that the mind, and hence consciousness, is a product of biological processes occurring in the brain, a reasonable next step is to consider molecules and circuits which may contribute to consciousness. There are numerous candidates; an investigator could "drop in" on a multitude of signaling hubs/networks which could, one day, inform the science of consciousness. Genes which function in multiple pathways impacting learning, memory, and emotions (including their dysregulation), are components of networks which plausibly underpin consciousness. Concentrating initially on a single or a few elements is admittedly reductionist, but this approach is often productive of larger insights.

⁙

IN THIS last section I will attempt to bind these recurring themes by offering an approach to the science of consciousness. There are numerous inspired theories, some more grounded in basic science than others. I agree with the perspective that the optimal opportunity to understand the contours of consciousness will happen when the neural circuitry, synapses, molecules, and cells that participate in the making of consciousness become known and functionally integrated. I also realize this goal may never be achieved. However, breakthroughs may come from unexpected directions. The results can potentially open a seam and suggest generative ways forward.

Since brain organoids will figure prominently in this discussion, it is appropriate to understand the appreciable limitations that currently exist. At present brain organoids can only be grown to a size of about 4 mm, a small structure. They contain about two to three million cells. An adult brain has about 85 billion neurons and a similar number of non-neural cells. Even though these organoids can be maintained in culture for up to two years,[110] they do not mature beyond the fetal or early newborn period. Many diseases have fetal origins and can be modeled, particularly disorders such as autism and microcephaly. Certain cell populations are sparse to absent, another limitation. For brain organoids these include, importantly, vascular and immune cells (microglia). Mesenchymal cells are sparse. For other organoids an absence of neurons is problematic, though obviously not for brain organoids. As detailed in the Microbes chapter, bacterial metabolites influence brain function. Thus far these elements have not been incorporated into the protocols. Improvements in all of these aspects of brain organoid generation are likely, though realistic expectations are warranted. Other limitations exist. We are aware of the importance of our senses and sense organs to our awareness. These no doubt play a large role in consciousness. How could brain organoids incorporate the contributions of sense organs? One group analyzed the diversity of cell types in brain organoids cultured for more than nine months. Included in the broad range of cells were retinal cells. The authors were able to control neuronal activity within the organoids using light stimulation of these light-responsive cells.[111] This is a start.

Even with these cautions and reservations a dialogue has opened, a dialogue which queries the notion, however remote this seems at present, that brain organoids could model consciousness, in effect "become conscious." Several studies have directed attention to this matter. One study was revelatory of the close link between brain organoid and preterm infant neural wiring.[112] Though there have been studies documenting similarity in organoid and human brain development at the cellular and molecular levels, there had been no evidence for the development of functional neural activity in organoids that was similar to that of human neurodevelopment prior to this study. Organoids grown for two months were recorded with a multi-electrode array. Excitatory glutamate and inhibitory GABA neurons were discerned. The recorded neural activity patterns were compared with the EEG (electroencephalogram) features of infants born prematurely

(24 to 38 weeks in this study). There were similarities at the network level. The authors suggest that this stable network activity may be genetically programmed. This study and others have fostered conferences, some partially sponsored by the NIH, devoted to speculations about the possibility of organoid consciousness and the looming ethical dimensions of organoid formation.[113, 114]

The idea of consciousness emanating from a brain organoid is a bridge considerably too far for most scientists at this time. We are leagues away from even an agreed upon definition of consciousness or how to measure it. Nonetheless, some serious scientists do not dismiss the possibility out of hand. A respected investigator in brain organoid research, Madeline Lancaster, provided an arresting quote for a recent article: "If you thought a fly was conscious, it's conceivable that an organoid could be".[115] Aside from the thought-stretching idea of organoid consciousness, the other side of this deliberative coin is the manner and extent to which we may utilize brain organoids to probe, at a minimum, a credible entry point into an exploration of consciousness. Facts beget facts; theories with scientific plausibility can emerge and be further tested.

At these early stages, intuition may play a necessary role. The intuition I have in mind is that fear can be marshalled to begin to explore consciousness. As noted in previous chapters, others have had similar intuitions. "Everyday" consciousness is phenomenal consciousness, that which can be verbally reported. Fear is a subjective, introspective state which can be articulated and which can serve as a basis for scientific studies, as in fear conditioning and fear memories. Fear conditioning may occur following a single trial and is difficult to extinguish. LeDoux and Damasio have argued that subjective, introspective states can be rigorously studied, as have others.[116] Fear, deeply embedded in the mind, is a reasonable starting point. This emotion is a component of anxiety, PTSD, phobias, and panic. As I and many others have experienced, panic is a stark manifestation of fear.

Creating "panic in a dish" is perhaps a reverie without merit, a meaningless metaphor. On the other hand, it may just be possible to engage the topic in a serious manner. Many scientists have considered other states as a basis to study consciousness, including epilepsy, anesthesia, sleep, loss of consciousness, and other conditions of impaired consciousness such as coma and persistent vegetative state. Investigations into these conditions entails studying consciousness by its absence. There is merit in this approach. Much can be learned by absence of function in biological systems. Panic, as I have subjectively reported herein, is also associated with a temporary abeyance of consciousness as we normally experience it. This is a discrete event which could potentially be modeled *in vitro*.

How might an investigator begin to study panic? I will suggest an approach, realizing it has flaws and may not pass muster at even a departmental seminar on new research ideas. However, one could conceive of studies with iPSC-derived brain organoids from persons with and without panic disorder. Minimizing genetic variation would provide more credible results. This would optimally involve genetically identical twins reared in the same household, as noted previously, one who experiences panic attacks and one who does not. Less ideal would be iPSC-derived organoids from brother Tim who does not have panic attacks and from me. We share fifty per cent of our genes. However, it has to be acknowledged at this primitive stage of the research that siblings discordant for panic would be far less ideal than monozygotic twin pairs, one with panic and his/her co-twin free of the disorder. As noted below, genetic alteration of stem cells used to grow brain organoids offers promise.

As implied by the foregoing, multiple protocols are available for organoid formation. For example, a forebrain structure could be derived, utilized by many of the studies I have cited. The forebrain gives rise to the majority of the human brain, including the neocortex, hippocampus, amygdala, and hypothalamus. It is likely all these structures, and others, participate in consciousness. A drawback, as noted, is the present state of developmental immaturity of these organoids. However, just as autism is a developmental disorder, it is reasonable to speculate that a trait as fundamental as consciousness would have origins in fetal life.

With this background in mind, we can contemplate the landscape of research possibilities. What might be studied which could provide a glimpse into a trait as daunting as consciousness? To initiate such an investigation, one could start with a focus on a gene such as ASIC1a, the gene which evokes neural transmission in an acid environment. An acidic environment could readily be created within the organoid. Not only has ASIC1a been implicated in panic, this protein is also implicated in learning and memory as previously noted. So ASIC1a—with myriad functions in learning and behavioral realms which are likely pillars in the structure of consciousness—is a reasonable candidate. There are surely many, many more. With acidification, one could study the proton gating properties of neurons in derived (or even fused) portions of an organoid, the effects on neurotransmission, and single cell RNA sequencing to determine changes in gene expression with changes in the experimental design. It is clear that large data bases from a diversity of cellular types in health and disease will greatly aid these studies, including proteomics, epigenomics, and others.[117] Additional routine and more sophisticated studies would be considered. Some of these are available, some are under development, and some have yet to be conceived. To be sure, even if one recorded a difference in an ASIC1a-mediated function between organoids from panic prone and panic resistant individuals, this may not tell us anything about consciousness. My goal has been to suggest an approach to consciousness, attempting to ground this or any approach one may consider on a solid basic science foundation.

Looking to the future, it will surely be the case that altering gene expression in brain organoids with gene editing tools such as CRISPR/Cas will play a large role in research involving consciousness. In parallel with gene editing, changes in the readouts of studies developed for the purpose of studying panic will be developed. Just as fear has left a discernible imprint, scientists may develop credible "panic assays."

⋮⋮⋮

THE FINAL chapter, like those before, has been inspired by mental phenomena which relate aspects of psychiatry to consciousness. The theme to be explored is reality, the bedrock of consciousness. Can the elements of reality be inserted into a basic science foundation of consciousness? The nature of reality is largely within the domain of physics, but no field of science is bounded by exclusivity. There is a place for persons like me who have lived a largely physics-averse life to try to meld the physical world with the mental. This may require a discussion of topics which many regard as fringe. To discuss reality also invites at least a modicum of philosophical musing. With these caveats, an attempt will be made to stay within an "acceptable" scientific frame.

CHAPTER FIVE

Reality
The Ultimate Arbiter of Consciousness

I AM TREADING INTO A MORASS of philosophical, physical, and psychological entanglements which may not, I fear, be clarifying, but which my lived experience compels me to engage with. The subject matter in this chapter title is heavily influenced by fleeting episodes in medical school, previously mentioned and fortunately uncommon, during which I had the disquieting sensation that what I was experiencing in the moment was not "real." The gestalt which felt very real was the "unreality" of the episodes. Though disturbed and confused, these experiences engendered intense curiosity about mental states such as these, leading to an impulse to learn more about what I now know is ontology, the broad branch of philosophy that studies reality. As implied above, reality has dimensions beyond the philosophical, including a psychological dimension and, as physicists and engineers know well, a physical dimension. Additionally, scholars from many disciplines studying consciousness also study ontology; bedrock reality and consciousness are inextricably linked. Psychology can be a bridge to demonstrate these linkages. Just as anxiety and depression may provide an entry point into consciousness via one of the most explicit manifestations of these disorders, panic, so too may these states of mind crack a window onto this most basic element of existence, consciousness, by a consideration of reality and a stark feeling of unreality.

These unsettling experiences are clearly delineated in the DSM V, psychiatry's latest Diagnostic and Statistical Manual. Within this manual is a description of Depersonalization/Derealization syndrome, the often co-mingled disturbances of the sense of self and of reality.[1] The cluster of symptoms characterizing the syndrome is the sense of detachment from oneself and surroundings, feelings of strangeness and disconnectedness. The borders between self and other become blurred. There may be, as noted, a powerful, distressing feeling of unreality. The disorders are also termed dissociative states. The waverings or fluctuations of consciousness can be fleeting with balance restored after a "mental scramble," creating a reality more in keeping with the affected person's baseline norm. Delusions or hallucinations are not a feature of the syndrome. An analysis of multiple studies (a meta-analysis) reveals that these altered states are commonly experienced at some point in an individual's lifetime.[2] In many cases there is associated trauma or abuse, inflating the numbers. Anxiety and depression are predisposing factors. About 1 to 2 percent of the population have the disorder on a chronic basis.[3]

When persons who experience Derealization/Depersonalization are asked to describe their symptoms, words are a poor means to convey the episode. The attempt is often couched in "as-if" language. "It feels as-if I were...."[4] The words expressing the sense of not being a participant in the usual interchanges of life are not adequate substitutes for the experience itself. However, it remains the case that these states are profoundly felt, despite an inability to articulate them. Persons experiencing these episodes retain insight and, again, exhibit no delusional ideation.

Episodes in an individual's life are often the impetus to delve deeper into a subject which previously may have been of passing interest. Derealization led to my surprise finding there was a field as seemingly obtuse as ontology. If not Reality, then what, Nothingness? Gottfried Leibniz, a German philosopher and polymath, posed this haunting question in the seventeenth century: Why is there Something rather than Nothing?[5] He would not, of course, have been the first to have considered, and perhaps been troubled by, this query. Philosophers and other scholars have given intellectual heft to this gnarly subject over many centuries. The abstraction is more than mere whimsy. We all have a consciousness of the great, often ineffable wonders of the universe; how did it come to be, what was there before, where does it end, how do I relate these imponderables to my existence? A goal in this chapter is to suggest some of the points of interchange which may link the mind, reality/consciousness, and the cosmos. A few of the putative connections may seem forced, but on a deep, experiential level I believe these links to be valid, to be compatible with some of the most creative theorizing on reality and consciousness.

Chapter 3 elaborated the use of optogenetics in mice to discern pathways involved in learning, memory, anxiety, and depression. The neuroanatomical basis of dissociative states has eluded description in the past. Remarkably, optogenetics in the murine species has also revealed a specific brain region and rhythm that produces a state in mice akin to dissociation observed in humans.[6] The authors of this study located a region in the mouse brain, the retrosplenial cortex, which responded to the drug ketamine—which is an antidepressant but also produces dissociation in humans—with the production of robust oscillations by electrical recording. When precise doses of ketamine were administered, this pattern of electrical activity was associated with dissociative-like behavior in the mice. They did not jump or rear up in response to threats and did not demonstrate escape movements when suspended by their tails. The responsible neurons were identified in layer 5 of the retrosplenial cortex. Additionally, an ion channel required for ketamine to elicit the behaviors indicative of dissociation was found. Light-sensing opsin proteins, one responsive to blue light producing neuronal stimulation and one responsive to yellow light producing inhibition, were directed to layer 5 neurons. Alternating blue and yellow light produced the same low frequency oscillations as did ketamine administration, resulting in the same dissociative-like behavior. Further, electrophysical recording demonstrated electrical coupling with the thalamus, but uncoupling from most other brain regions.

This same study involved a patient with epilepsy whose aura prior to a seizure included dissociation. Electrodes were implanted in various regions to determine the focus of these auras heralding a seizure. This is standardly done in clinical practice and has been a boon to researchers. Stimulation of the deep posteromedial cortex, homologous to the murine retrosplenial cortex, produced the same brain rhythm seen in the mice, accompanied by a self-reported dissociative experience. The commonality of results identifies the biological substratum for a cortical rhythm that defines states of dissociation. Sophisticated studies such as this one assist in understanding altered states of consciousness at a basic level.

⋄⋄⋄

A STUDY of reality must incorporate what we understand about the physical world and its origin. Our interconnected reality extends from the tiniest particles of the quantum world to the vastness of the known universe. In the early 1900s, when Albert Einstein was completing his work on the general theory of relativity, the universe was considered to be static, consisting of a single galaxy, our Milky Way, beyond which there existed a dark, empty, unchanging void. Two major discoveries revealed not a static universe, but one characterized by dynamism. No scenario could be more dynamic than the origin of the universe. All credible evidence has indicated that it began as the Big Bang (a facetious term coined by Fred Hoyle), an unimaginably tiny, hot, and dense speck that burst into existence 13.8 billion years ago,[7] unleashing the fundamental elements and forces creating all things animate and inanimate.

A second finding which illustrates the dynamism of the universe was the observation attributed to Edwin Hubble in the 1920s that the universe was expanding.[8] The studies from his group provided evidence for an expanding universe by noting that the wavelengths of light from stars called Cepheid variables, whose pattern of brightness provided a means to determine distance from Earth, were redshifted (longer) than expected for a static universe, indicating movement of these stars away from observers on Earth. This is analogous to the Doppler effect for sound waves; i.e., the higher pitch of a siren moving toward an observer (due to a compressive effect on the sound waves) and reduced pitch (lengthened sound waves) after the siren passes. Hubble was able to link distances of these stars with their redshift patterns, showing that Cepheid variables of distant galaxies recede more rapidly than closer ones, the definition of an expanding universe.

Lest there had been lingering doubt concerning the validity of the Big Bang as currently conceived, the investigations of John Mather and George Smoot, work for which they won the Nobel Prize in 2006, provided ample documentation. Radiation remaining from the Big Bang had been detected in the 1960s, though its wavelength had become stretched to the microwave range. This heat is now known as the cosmic microwave background (CMB), early remnants of the Big Bang. Using instrumentation aboard a NASA satellite, the Mather group recorded the spectrum of the microwaves constituting the CMB that accorded with expectations based on Big Bang cosmology.[9] The Smoot team demonstrated slight temperature fluctuations in this pervasive afterglow of the Big Bang, a signature of clumps of matter in the infant universe destined to become stars and galaxies.[10]

In the earliest fraction of a second following the Big Bang the universe inflated dramatically and has been expanding and cooling since. The first elements were dominated by helium and hydrogen. When the universe had cooled sufficiently these gases coalesced to form the first stars roughly 400 million years after the Big Bang. Stars are born and they die. At the end of this cycle, some become sufficiently hot to forge heavier elements like carbon, calcium, oxygen, and iron as one element fuses into another, heavier element by nucleosynthesis, ending in a thermonuclear explosion, widely scattering these elements and allowing the existence of living matter. In Carl Sagan's oft-quoted dictum, "we are all star dust."

These explosions enabled the discovery of another startling fact. The expansion of the universe is *accelerating*. This finding relied upon the selection of a "standard candle" of invariant brightness, coupled with measurement of the redshift of the light from these receding, luminous objects which had exploded. These were utilized by Saul Perlmutter, Brian Schmidt, and Adam Reiss, all awarded a Nobel Prize in 2011 for their discoveries.[11, 12] To achieve their results, they needed to see deeper into space (closer in time to the Big Bang) to find and maximize information from the optimal standard candles, including detailed knowledge of its light spectrum. This capability was provided by the Hubble Space Telescope with its battery of large electronic cameras. Their standard candle was the result of rare thermonuclear explosions, cited in the previous paragraph, of a category of star called a supernova type 1a. When these stars reach a critical mass and explode, the brilliance is often more than the combined brightness of all the stars in the galaxy of which they are a part. The redshift they detected was greater than what would be expected for an expanding, but non-accelerating universe. Calculations suggest the expansion of the universe has been accelerating for billions of years.

Robert Kirschner, thesis advisor for Schmidt and Reiss who started both on the paths to their discoveries, wrote an engaging story of the search for type 1a supernovae and the demanding science required to maximize their value as standard candles, the great utility of newer instruments such as the Hubble Telescope capable of penetrating deep space, the struggle to schedule time on this and other, land-based telescopes, and the intriguing personalities and competition motivating these quests.[13] The sighting of an explosion (estimated at only one to two per galaxy per century) set off a scramble to collect the requisite information. More than an exposition on exploding stars and cosmic acceleration, the Kirschner book demonstrated how two investigative streams, information from supernovae and temperature fluctuations in the CMB, intersected to help substantiate not only the age, but also the composition of the universe.

Two mysterious substances form the bulk of the universe, dark energy and dark matter. Dark energy constitutes approximately 68 percent, dark matter 27 percent, and ordinary matter 5 percent of the universe. Dark energy and dark matter are forces known by their purported effects rather than direct observation. There have been several lines of investigation, including those of Mather and Smoot, indicating there is more mass with its gravitational effect than previously acknowledged. Dark matter is thought to fill this void. Dark energy is thought to be the counteracting force ("pushing outward"), sustaining an expanding universe. This raises the question of whether dark energy is continually added as the accelerated expansion continues. Scientists would like to know much more about these forces, including the particle(s) constituting these entities. The photon, for example carries the force of electromagnetism, and there is currently an active search for the graviton, the postulated force-carrying particle of gravity. These and many other unknowns fuel our fascination (and dread) when we study and contemplate the universe, including the possibility of extra (hidden or unobserved) dimensions, and gruesome scenarios depicting the cessation of the universe.[14]

Conversely, the picture is filling in for the world of the very tiny, the quantum world. The Standard Model (SM) represents all the fundamental interactions underpinning the formation of stars, galaxies, planets and, ultimately, living matter. The elements of the Standard Model, leptons, quarks, and a multitude of other particles, have been prised from the fabric of matter by decades of brilliant theorizing and experimentation. The remaining fixture of the SM, the Higgs boson (a boson is a force-carrying particle), was postulated to exist decades ago by a Scottish physicist, Peter Higgs,[15] and five other scientists. The conviction that this particle could be fleetingly captured led to the construction of the Large Hadron Collider (LHC), a 16-mile underground track on the Swiss-French border. A huge magnet propels oppositely traveling beams of protons at energies far exceeding the capabilities of other accelerators. When the protons smash together, the scatter of particles resulting from these collisions can be analyzed. Two teams, each using a different detector, announced in the summer of 2012 they had clear evidence for the existence of the Higgs boson.[16, 17] Following the success at the LHC, Higgs and François Englert were awarded Nobel Prizes. The LHC has been upgraded and will be operating at higher energies, with the expectation that other particles will be discovered.

The overriding significance of the Higgs boson is that it provides the mechanism to transmit mass to the other particles. The photon, which has remained massless, is the lone exception. The Higgs boson has been variously described as a virtual particle, a vibration, or an excited ripple in the Higgs field that occupies the vacuum of space. The theoretical physicist Sean Carroll has provided a lucid story of the search for the Higgs boson and explanation of the Higgs field.[18] This field can be likened to a viscous fluid which retards the motion of the other particles, thereby imparting mass. The more a given particle interacts with the field, the greater its mass. It is the Higgs boson that gives the Higgs field its properties. Carroll relates this field to the other fields which surround us and to the intricacies (and mysteries) of quantum field theory. Fields of multiple, different physical descriptions pervade the universe, including the electromagnetic and gravitational fields. Particles, like the photon which carries electromagnetism, are tiny vibrations in these fields.

The provision of mass within the first fraction of a second following the Big Bang represented a dramatic phase transition, a change in matter mentioned in the last chapter. Phase transitions are accompanied by a loss of symmetry, a property inherent to the laws of Nature. Symmetry resists change; it remains unaltered by time or location or position of the observer.[19] Nobel laureate Frank Wilczek has described symmetry as Change Without Change in his illuminating book on Nature's designs.[20] Symmetries can be broken, as was referenced when describing stem cells in previous Chapters. A pluripotent cluster of embryonic stem cells can lose symmetry spontaneously, as when a subset of these cells self-organizes to form beating cardiac tissue with no outside intervention. Embryonic stem cells also break symmetry when defined chemicals are added to direct the cells down a chosen developmental pathway.

As Carroll has emphasized, symmetries help to inform our understanding of deep processes. The breaking of symmetries is also highly instructive.

Powerful symmetries gave rise to the four fundamental forces of Nature following the Big Bang—the strong nuclear force which holds the atom's nucleus together, the weak nuclear force, gravity, and electromagnetism. These forces arose following instances of symmetry breaking. Symmetries, symmetry breaking, and the subsequent patterns are the hidden regularities of Nature. A marvelous example of hidden regularities is the ordering of the elements, manufactured in stars and scattered widely across the universe by their explosions. These coalesced into the Periodic Table.[21] This exquisite pattern was recognized by the Russian Dmitri Mendeleev. Though overlooked in life, his contribution was finally recognized 50 years after his death when the 101st element of the Periodic Table was named mendelevium.

The foregoing hints at the behaviors of the tiny that give form to our larger world, the existence we consider our reality. But this realm is baffling and bizarre. As one example of many, quantum particles can pass through impenetrable barriers via quantum tunnelling. Measurements in the observable Newtonian or classical world can be considered reliable, subject only to the exactitude one wishes to impose. But quantum measurements are inherently uncertain; e.g., the position *and* momentum of a particle cannot be known. If the position is known, the momentum cannot be known, and vice-versa. Interacting particles also become "entangled." Their interaction produces a state wherein knowledge of a property—like spin or charge of one particle—assures knowledge of the spin or charge of its entangled partner, no matter their separation. Prior to observation, the particles are in a superposition of possible states. A Chinese study has shown entanglement of partners separated by greater than 700 miles.[22] Einstein labeled this "spooky action at a distance," and opined that some deeper principle of physics, yet unknown, would provide an explanation. So much about quantum mechanics is unusual, mystifying really, which led Nobel laureate Richard Feynman to declare that "I think I can safely say that no one understands quantum mechanics."[23]

Despite the difficulties in comprehending quantum mechanics, a focus on the basics is paramount. As particle physicist and Nobel laureate Leon Lederman attests, the objective of his field is "…to identify the primordial particles of nature—those from which all nature is made—and codify the laws of physics that oversee their properties and *social* (italics added) behavior."[24] Sean Carroll reserves a central role for particle physics when he proclaims that "we are part of the universe. Everything in the human body is successfully described by the Standard Model of particle physics.... Knowing that our atoms obey the Standard Model isn't very helpful when it comes to real-world problems of politics, psychology, economics, or romance; but any ideas you have along those lines must at least conform to what we know about the behavior of elementary particles."[18] (p. 280)

⁝⁝⁝

WITH A murky understanding of the quantum, it seems unlikely that we might fully understand how this realm became the recognizable world we inhabit any time soon. It is appropriate to note that Darwinian principles, the guiding heuristic in the biological sphere, have been applied to a wide range of phenomena, including the quantum to classical transition. The Darwinian process in the living world is one of natural selection acting upon spontaneously arising genetic variants to favor those variants with the highest survival and reproductive potential. Some theorists believe a similar dynamic (quantum Darwinism) has been at work to construct our observable world from its fundamental particles. A leading figure in this endeavor is Wojeciech Zurek, a theoretical physicist whose mentor was John Wheeler (more about him in this chapter). The argument raised by Zurek and his colleagues posits that certain states of the vast possible arrangement of particles are more stable and can be selected in preference to less stable arrangements.[25] This iterated process leads to persistence of these selected patterns in the familiar, classical world. Lawrence Krauss, a theoretical physicist and cosmologist, has stressed that "quantum mechanical systems explore all possible trajectories, even those that are classically forbidden, as they evolve in time."[26] (p. 161)

At this juncture, it is reasonable to return to a version of the question posed by Leibniz: how did we get from Nothing to Something? Providing even the barest outline requires a continuing appeal to the counterintuitive. Lawrence Krauss has offered a view on the process which could have plausibly led to the world we inhabit from Nothing (empty space in his words).[26] The vacuum of space, once thought to be devoid of energy and particles, is known to have both negative and positive energy and to be a seething, vibrating mix of virtual particles popping into and out of existence on minuscule time scales. Krauss offers the logic that quantum fluctuations at the beginning produced slight asymmetries—the key one being a slight excess of matter over antimatter. These fluctuations later became the matter of the universe, reflected in the cosmic microwave background. His conclusion: Nothing is unstable. Krauss credits Frank Wilczek as the first to state that Nothing is unstable.[27] At the beginning, as Wilczek has similarly related, there may have been a true vacuum with a co-existing state of undisturbed symmetry. A phase transition producing less symmetry could have appeared and expanded rapidly, releasing energy and resulting in the formation of particles and ultimately the universe; the reason there is Something rather than Nothing is that Nothing is unstable.

How are we to think of reality as a philosophical and psycho-physical construct? What is real? The search for the quiddity, the essence of existence is a rich intellectual pursuit. A daughter-father team has written a delightful book of serious scholarship on this matter.[28] A principal aim was to explicate the writings and musings of John Archibald Wheeler, a towering figure in twentieth-century physics. He mentored many leading physicists of the day, some of whom were interviewed by Amanda Gefter and her father. Wheeler left us with a concept of the universe as a "self-excited circuit;" the universe creating a mammal with a brain capable of creating reality, and this mammal peering back to its attachment to the Big Bang, the whole a self-sustaining, causal loop.[29] Wheeler coined the term "it from bit," and with it a conviction that information is fundamental to the matrix of reality. He had a deep sense that the quantum was at the core and that observership (through measurement in the quantum realm) was key to assembling the information that stoked the self-excited circuit. The Gefters pored over the deliberations of this man driven to determine how reality is constructed. These were kept in notebooks which resided in the library of the American Philosophical Society. Wheeler stressed a participatory universe—that observers are intrinsic to the process. In these journals he sought the role consciousness may play, though with no resolution. He often invoked Charles Darwin in his deliberations. He believed that the structure of the universe was connected with our existence in a fundamental way. He struggled with the inside/ outside dichotomy, whether observations/reality were embedded within or imposed from without, referred to as the God's-eye view.

In this book the Gefters also reviewed the work of theoretical physicist Carlo Rovelli.[30, 31] He noted that distinct observers do not report the same information when presented a sequence of events. His work, which argues against the prevailing view that reality exists apart from observers, revealed that properties and measurements within quantum mechanics are *relative* to a given observer, that systems are *relational*. His conclusion is that the nature of reality is observer dependent, altering the commonly held perspective. When Rovelli was interviewed for the book, he credited Wheeler's notion that information was the right concept, which structured his own conclusions about reality.

Rovelli's work was instrumental for the conclusions the Gefters ultimately drew. They had posed for themselves the same intellectual challenge Wheeler had ardently pursued: what, when plumbed at depth, is reality? Their insights, in part, were these: Nothing is an invariant feature with symmetry, and therefore contains little information; asymmetry creates information. The quantum, determined through exhaustive experimentation to provide a reliable description of the world, is at the core. Each observer creates an observer dependent reality when their measurements in the quantum break the symmetry and produce reality-creating information. The primary insight is that reality is observer dependent, radically so as Rovelli had asserted. Reality-creation comes from inside, not outside. These conclusions may seem fringe, even indecipherable/unfathomable. I share this bewilderment but would defend the notion that this deep dive into the essence of reality is the type of inquiry which usefully stretches the boundaries of this dialogue. As the great polymath J. B. S. Haldane asserted: "My own suspicion is that the universe is not only queerer than we suppose, but queerer than we *can* suppose."[32]

⸭⸭⸭

I HAVE a friend from childhood. He was also an end on our high school football team. During this time, he was a perfectionist in the most painful sense of the word. He was constantly, in his view, falling short of the expectations he imposed on himself. Ron became a dentist. Fortunately for his patients, he continued to set high standards. Fortunately for him, his barrage of personal punishment ended when he became a practitioner of meditation in the tradition of Eastern philosophy. I envy the peace he has found. He leads groups in the principles and practice of his chosen way to access this inner tranquility. I have visited him often over the past few decades.

Conveniently, he lives in Colorado near a ski area. After a day on the slopes, our conversation often turns to the weighty subjects of meditation and consciousness. How are we to regard these? When Ron meditates, he feels he is accessing a realm apart from his material mind, though the tranquility is sensed internally. These discussions always suggested the dualist/materialist distinction, to be discussed, which has long represented the spectrum of views on consciousness. Admittedly, Ron and I did not make deep inroads into the subject matter, but the effort was meaningful to us.

I am persuaded that the locus of reality creation is "inside." Reality is a physical construct as well as a personal, experiential one. We have followed a portion of the scholarship that has shown a path from Nothing to Something. We have reviewed the line of reasoning that indicates observers create their own reality. If reality creation is internal, it seems reasonable to assert that an individual mind in distress may deconstruct that reality, experiencing a sense of estrangement, the profound sense that reality feels unreal. If we are the architects of our radically observer dependent reality, isn't it that reality which is splintered or fragmented in the context of Derealization? In one's construction of the world, there may be cracks in the foundation and chipping at the margins. These builders are the ones whose genetic constitution and environment have predisposed them to periodically cross some threshold, entering a temporarily altered reality. If we understood these phenomena at a deeper, physical level we may gain special insight into consciousness, our awareness of ourselves and our surroundings, our reality.

It will challenge credulity to assert that individuals create their reality from internal sources, incorporating quantum building blocks. The general outline is provocative, but details which are generally accepted by the scientific community are wanting at this time. Within this context, however, it is appropriate to note that many scholars use the term "construction" or "assembly" or "making" when speaking of aspects of consciousness. Components which feed into consciousness, such as emotions, are conceived to be constructed entities by Lisa Barrett, referenced in Chapter 4. She is well known for her theory of constructed emotion.[33] Joseph LeDoux, cited multiple times in the last chapter, offers the view that emotions are cognitively assembled states of autonoietic consciousness,[34] human consciousness able to place a self in the past or future. Memories, another key contributor to consciousness, are also conceived as constructed entities by some scholars. Brains construct meaning and govern action from experience and the senses. For the psychologist Daniel Schacter, an important function of memory is to allow individuals to simulate or imagine future episodes. This requires a system that can flexibly draw on the past and recombine elements of experience. [35, 36]

⁂

IF YOU stretch your imagination, Nothingness might serve as a metaphor for Derealization; so too might Infinity be a metaphor for Depersonalization, a state in which boundaries are blurred. No boundary engenders more astonishment and, for some, fear, than contemplation of the ultimate boundary, Infinity.[37] Blaise Pascal, a seventeenth-century physicist and philosopher, allowed that "the silence of infinite space terrified me."[38] For the Jewish philosopher Martin Buber, contemplation of infinity evoked a reaction of utter despair: "A necessity I could not imagine swept over me: I had to try again and again to imagine the edge of space, or its edgelessness, time with a beginning and an end or time without a beginning or end, and both were equally impossible, equally hopeless…. Under an irresistible compulsion I reeled from one to the other, at times so closely threatened with the danger of madness that I seriously thought of avoiding it by suicide."[39]

⁂

SENSORY SYSTEMS figure prominently when lay people or professionals think of consciousness. The principal senses are vision, hearing, smell, taste, and sound. On a reduced scale, vision represents the complexity that consciousness represents on a large scale. Different cells and pathways respond to the features of vision; motion, depth, edges, form, color. The broad outline of the steps the brain utilizes in constructing visual images is known, but the details which allow the integration of all these features into an integrated whole, the binding problem, is an area of intense study. The binding problem of vision is a model for the binding problem of consciousness writ large, the requirement that consciousness knit together all the disparate elements of which we are aware in the ongoing moments in time. Indeed, two leading consciousness researchers, Christof Koch and Francis Crick (now decreased), have utilized the visual system as a framework, a scheme for what they conceive (and study) as the neural correlates of visual consciousness.[40] They have reasoned that success in this endeavor can be a model for the vastly larger project of understanding consciousness.

There are also studies of non-sensory capabilities which inform us about the structure of neural systems interacting with the environment. For example, there are "face" cells which fire in response to facial visualization, and "mirror neurons" in observers which mimic the firing pattern of the same cells of individuals performing a task. For decades there has been research, much of it in the rat, focused on the intriguing organization of our internally generated representations of space and time. These, in turn, are integrated in the hippocampus as episodic memories are formed.[41] Two key cells within the spatial system are the "grid" cells in the entorhinal cortex which project to the hippocampus and form a pattern of firing representing space, and "place" cells within the hippocampus which fire whenever a rat is in a certain location.[42] To these basic cell types have been added "time" cells, a population of lateral entorhinal cortex neurons which project to the hippocampus.[43] The ability of these cells to encode episodic time may be integrated with spatial information from the medial entorhinal cortex. These may, in turn, be integrated into a unified representation of what, when, and where. These representations may then be stored by the hippocampus.[44]

An intriguing philosophical excursion is offered by the ability of the brain to represent space and time. Immanuel Kant, an eighteenth-century German philosopher, believed that there are two innate intuitions, space and time, which structure the entirety of our experience.[45] Two studies tested the idea that one of these universals, space, is already in place before an animal leaves its nest to encounter its external environment, that is before it can learn its surroundings. Both groups were able to implant electrodes into the hippocampus of 14-day-old, freely moving rat pups, and record activity of neurons at 16 days, only two days after eye opening. Both groups showed that place cells and another neuronal subtype, head-direction neurons, were functional at this time, arguing that spatial cognitive abilities are inherent. The senior authors of these two studies, John O'Keefe[46] and Edvard and May-Britt Moser,[47] have produced substantial knowledge of the cells and neural circuits in the hippocampus and surrounding structures which allow us to navigate our environments. The space and temporal functions of these circuits are thought to be the organizing elements for remembered events. For their work, these three investigators were awarded a Nobel Prize in

2014. Sensory systems, exemplified by vision, and non-sensory processes, represented by space and time, must be accounted for in any robust theory of consciousness.

⁝⁝⁝

IN 2018 I went to the Science of Consciousness conference in Tucson, held annually since 1994. I wanted to get a sense for the range of scholarship impacting consciousness. The spectrum was vast. There were numerous presentations by leaders in the field which were scientifically rigorous. There were many poster presentations which were quasi-scientific, exploring the links between consciousness and meditation practice, mystical experiences, and related spheres. Currently, those who have staked out consciousness as their focus find themselves in a big-tent community.

I was paying particular attention to talks and posters at the conference which might indicate the extent to which quantum mechanics has entered the consciousness dialogue. I had read another book in the finest tradition of interview, interspersed with the author's finely wrought and deeply considered insights, Jim Holt's *Why Does the World Exist?* [48] One of his interviewees was Sir Roger Penrose (knighted in 1994 by Queen Elizabeth). His knowledge of physics and mathematics is legendary, as is his prodigious literary output. He received a Nobel Prize in 2020 for mathematically demonstrating that Einstein's general theory of relativity was a strong predictor of black hole formation. Penrose has been a leading proponent of the claim that quantum processes must be the basis of consciousness. His arguments are most forcibly made in his book *Shadows of the Mind*. [49] The quantum, postulated by Penrose and others to underlie the neural processes supporting the coherence or bundling of our ongoing consciousness, are the "shadows" alluded to in the book's title, the hidden coordinators of conscious thought. Penrose spoke at the Tucson conference, but I confess the material was difficult to grasp. Though impressions are suspect, there was certainly a segment of the audience either skeptical or outright hostile to a role for quantum mechanics. The traditional dogma, to which most scientists hold fast, asserts that biological processes are best explained in the "classical" realm without the need for quantum mechanics. Neuroscience is typically viewed as the most productive avenue for investigating consciousness.

As the particles, forces, and fields of the universe are being scrutinized, gravity has still not been accommodated into a unified theory. Einstein's theory of relativity beautifully weaves space and time into a four-dimensional fabric known as spacetime—which is how we understand gravity. Gravity warps spacetime. The general theory of relativity appears to be incompatible with quantum mechanics. Unifying the two to construct a quantum theory of gravity remains one of the major challenges confronting physics. The problem has also impacted the thinking of Penrose. He believes an understanding of consciousness would be facilitated if physicists could unite quantum mechanics with the classical world via a validated theory of quantum gravity.

⁝⁝⁝

MUCH OF the foregoing begs the question whether quantum mechanics explains some aspects of biology. If this was to be the case, this would lend some credence to possible involvement of quantum mechanics within the consciousness sphere. A relatively small group of investigators is beginning to answer this in the affirmative. For instance, quantum mechanics may explain some aspects of enzyme action and the sense of smell.[50] Mention has been made in Chapter 2 that the shuttling of electrons through the respiratory chain in mitochondria may involve quantum processes.[51] Quantum mechanics has been demonstrated in the life sustaining process of photosynthesis. There is direct evidence that rapid energy transfer, a consequence of photon capture by light-harvesting complexes in photosynthesizing microorganisms, is accomplished via quantum transport.[52]

A particularly compelling example of quantum involvement is magnetoreception, the ability of a migrating animal to utilize the Earth's weak magnetic field to travel long distances. Diverse species of animals, from birds and fishes to insects, depend upon magnetoreception.[53] How animals sense the magnetic field and use it as a compass has been an enigma, though it had been postulated that this field likely influences a chemical reaction. Previous work had pointed to magnetically sensitive proteins called cryptochromes located in the retina. Certain cryptochromes are involved in the regulation of circadian rhythms. A group has now shown that a cryptochrome subtype, cryptochrome 4, shows magnetic sensitivity in the night-migrating European robin.[54] The research, revealing involvement of quantum spin dynamics of electrons, was carried out *in vitro*. Nonetheless, this work is quite close to revealing how the magnetic properties of a field can interact with molecules able to sense this field to aid spatial orientation and migration. Quantum compasses may be more prevalent in Nature than we have realized.

Some investigators like Roger Penrose, noting the role of the quantum realm in non-classical biological processes as cited above, argue that quantum mechanics is necessary for the speed and coherence required of consciousness. It seems reasonable that a starting point to assess speed and coherence might be neuronal firing and synaptic transmission, generating the multiple functions we associate with brain activity.[55] An action potential initiates the extremely rapid and selective flow of ions across the nerve cell membrane as the spike travels down the nerve. It is possible these ion channels could maintain their coherence via quantum mechanical processes like entanglement. Even if there is quantum entanglement locally (within a single neuron), a mental activity such as a thought must be coordinated across a large portion of the brain. Decoherence would likely follow, leading to a default, classical state. There are interesting speculations regarding how brain-wide coherence may be accomplished. One theory relates that there could be quantum interaction between the electromagnetic field, which pervades the brain and is generated by the electrical activity of its nerves, and the voltage which opens and closes these voltage-gated ion channels.[50] (p. 267–8) There is presently no evidence for quantum mechanical processes in the generation of consciousness, but this will be a fascinating arena to follow.

⸪

IT IS HARD to broach the topic of consciousness without discussing the spectrum of approaches from materialism to dualism. In the materialist view, brain and mind are not separable from the remainder of the body. They function as an integrated biological whole. We have encountered Derek Denton previously who expressed the materialist view in a straightforward manner: "The mind, which has for centuries been considered as the incorporeal subject of all psychical faculties and often been severed from the body that houses it, isn't a separate entity, but quite simply and definitively what the brain does."[56] In these early days when consciousness remains an enigma, theories abound. LeDoux has listed 20 contemporary theories of consciousness and their proponents which have a physicalist/materialist basis.[34] (p. 273) For materialists, consciousness will ultimately be shown to result from physico-chemical processes in the brain, explained under the broad rubric of neuroscience. Many materialists are actively researching the neural correlates of consciousness (NCC), defined as the minimum neural mechanisms jointly sufficient for a specific conscious experience,[57] such as visual perception. In contradistinction, dualism transports consciousness beyond the material body. The French philosopher René Descartes proclaimed that consciousness fell outside the rules that govern other aspects of the physical world, that it was a fundamental property which has no spatial dimension, whereas the body exists in both space and time. Descartes was a dualist. Dualists have traditionally equated consciousness with the soul.

From what I have written thus far, particularly in Chapter 4, it appears I have committed to the materialist camp. That would, in general, be the case. There may, however, be a view of consciousness which merits consideration (see below) that can bridge some of the problems scholars have had with both materialism and dualism. To reiterate, materialism is the thesis that the physical state of one's mind *is* consciousness. Critics of materialism argue that these physical states representing consciousness cannot explain the subjective experiences people report: sensory experiences, emotions, and thoughts. These are the so-called qualia of experience, the redness and smell of a rose and the delight these evoke. Materialism cannot answer the reasons/mechanisms for subjective qualities. This has famously been termed "the hard problem" of consciousness.[58] Dualism, on the other hand, suffers from the fact that there is no evidence of causal effects in the brain owing to any form of nonphysical input, and is therefore rejected by most scientists. It is notable that several consciousness scholars, including David Chalmers who originated the "hard problem" conundrum, hold a position called naturalistic dualism. The immaterial mind, in this view, is not a mystical entity, but a part of Nature, subject to the same laws and principles. Naturalistic dualism illustrates the range of thinking impacting consciousness.

As noted, both materialism and dualism have explanatory impediments. Is there a philosophical strain which could fill the explanatory gap? One candidate which has attained a measure of academic respectability is panpsychism, the notion that every component of the physical world has consciousness, graded from extremely rudimentary, including particles like electrons, to complex. Philip Goff has lucidly elaborated the philosophy of panpsychism,[59] building upon the scholarship of early twentieth-century astronomer Arthur Eddington[60] and philosopher and Nobel laureate Bertrand Russell.[61] Physical science tells us what elements of the physical world do, how they behave. The argument for panpsychism is that constituents of the physical world have an *intrinsic* nature apart from the dictates of physical science. This intrinsic nature, as the argument goes, encompasses consciousness. To be credible, one must hold the view that consciousness could exist within the intrinsic nature of materials in the universe and be pervasive in the sense that fields, spacetime, and electromagnetism are pervasive. Even these entities are characterized by the physics community by what they do based on measurement. Physical science does not seek information on intrinsic natures. On the surface, panpsychism seems absurd. However, for anyone interested in consciousness, the effort to understand panpsychism will be repaid.

Panpsychism, so the argument goes, reaches its highest level of organization in the consciousness of humans after billions of years of evolution. Atomic and subatomic particles could have rudimentary bits of consciousness, as noted. As these and other particles are combined and recombined in an infinitude of ways, consciousness evolving toward that in humans appears, though where along this path the experience of consciousness arises is, of course, not known. Simple forms of consciousness, existing as features of the material world, are put forward as fundamental for the attainment of complex consciousness.

Panpsychism is tied to the same combination or binding problem which bedevils any theory of consciousness. Goff cites two principal lines of investigation which are being pursued to attempt to determine how panpsychism could solve this. One tack would assess the prospect that emergence, a concept raised in foregoing chapters, could help explain the development of increasingly complex consciousness based on fundamental principles of Nature. A second strategy would be a reductionist one, supplying an explanation for how complex forms of consciousness can be successively built from simpler forms. This is akin to the constructive processes of emotion and memory formation referenced previously, though the putative building blocks are of a more fundamental nature. Progress will be slow and uncertain, but Goff provides an apt analogy: "Just as it took a century working within the Darwinian paradigm to get to DNA, so it will require decades or centuries of interdisciplinary labor to fill in the details of Russell-Eddington panpsychism."[59] (p. 175)

Goff confesses that his passion is ontology, as is the case for many who study consciousness. Panpsychism is a theory of reality; reality underpins consciousness. Panpsychism has intellectual appeal. I question, however, if it has a separate lane between materialism and dualism. Materialists believe that a brain state *is* the consciousness one experiences, not that the brain produces consciousness. I can conceive that consciousness is a pervasive, intrinsic feature of the natural order. I can also conceive that integrated consciousness is instantiated in the building blocks from elementary particles to chemistry and physics to the material structures of neuroscience. So, possibly, the panpsychism lane, if it exists, is merged with the materialist lane? I am sympathetic with the views of others I have referenced that the elementary particles of quantum mechanics must have a foundational role.

One of the remaining great mysteries is the origin of life. This was another threshold with, perhaps, quantum involvement. A series of lectures by Erwin Schrödinger, physicist and Nobel laureate, was published in 1944 under the title *What is Life?*[62] He maintained that quantum mechanics played a major role. Paul Davies argues that to have gotten life started, information would have needed to be replicated. This can be accomplished at vastly greater speeds by quantum processes such as superposition, entanglement, and tunneling than can possibly be accomplished by classical processes. The nature of an information replicator is unknown, but "once a population of information replicators became established, quantum uncertainty provided an inbuilt mechanism for variation. Throw in a selection mechanism and the great darwinian (*sic*) game could begin."[63] If this general theme is correct (a big if), it is not a stretch to imagine that the quantum realm could have undergirded the molecular realm, and that selected combinatorial variations could have led to more complex forms of life cobbled from simpler forms.

⁂

I BEGAN this chapter with experiences of unreality. These experiences and curiosity led to a desire to try as comprehensively as I might to understand reality and the physical manner by which it might intersect with and support consciousness. I am persuaded by the arguments which situate reality in the "inner space" of individual minds, and that extremes of psycho-physical states of mind can profoundly impact reality and consciousness. If our minds are central to reality, and by extension consciousness, then it is logical to assume minds are central to the disassembly/deconstruction which can occur in states of distress. In my view, these are not states of mind imported from without.

Though we all experience disorder at times in our lives, often extreme, and are wobbled by these experiences, most individuals emerge with their desire to engage their fellow humans and the world intact. This desire to engage can extend to the universe. Among our most significant successes in space have been the Voyager 1 and Voyager 2 missions, mentioned in the personal narrative. These were launched in 1977 to explore the outer planets, Jupiter, Saturn, Uranus, and Neptune, at a propitious time when these giants were clustered on one side of the sun, allowing a facilitated fly-by to accomplish their proposed studies. Exploration of these planets was the mission, but with ingenuity and a modest budget, project managers urged the robots further and further. It was reported that Voyager 1 crossed into interstellar space beyond our solar system in the summer of 2012,[64] still sending data back to Earth. Subsequently, Voyager 2 has also transited our solar system.

Jim Bell chronicled the Voyager mission. As he writes, "mission directors were eager to directly measure the interstellar fields, particles, and waves beyond the influence of the sun. In other words, to extend the reach of human senses into interstellar space."[65] This desire to extend the reach of human senses found poignant expression in the Carl Sagan-inspired messages from Earth placed aboard the Voyager probes. These were gold-plated copper phonograph records, onto which were etched musical selections, audio messages in over 50 languages, and over 100 images of the Earth, along with instructions for retrieving and interpreting these various forms of human communication. Though the chance intelligent life would find and comprehend the contents of these Golden Records on the two Voyager probes is minuscule, the attempt to extend our humanity is a telling feature of the human condition.

Owing to evolutionary dynamics, we possess the consciousness to conceive sending Golden Records into space. From but a twig on a branch of the tree of life, the human race is nonetheless in the uniquely privileged position to cast a reflective view backward and project into the future, to mine the past in an attempt to build an intellectual edifice onto which future investigations from many disciplines may be added which will impact our understanding of consciousness. That there are truths yet to be revealed which will yield to our species' restless, incessant probing is the promise. Some of these insights will wedge a door, even permit entry into heretofore dark passageways, shuttered rooms, and locked closets of Nature's most deeply sequestered secrets.

Acknowledgments

WRITING IS A CHALLENGE. I am indebted to those with whom I shared this work and whose opinions I knew would be credible and honest. Their encouragement has aided me greatly. The book would not have been published without a fortuitous encounter with Holly Carver, former Director of the University of Iowa Press. In a city touted for its writing programs, Holly is well known and respected for the generous help she provides to aspiring writers. She not only reviewed a segment of writing I had done but invited me to join a local science book club. Another member of this club, Sara T. Sauers, owns a publication design business. The book has been published with her essential help. I thank Kitty Chibnik for her meticulous compilation of the index.

Tim and Marilyn read chapter 1 and offered encouragement. I particularly thank Nancy Wyland, an MFA graduate of the University of Iowa, who lent her considerable writing skills to the personal narrative over cups of coffee before the pandemic outbreak. Karen Williams, a high school classmate, was an early supporter and astute reader of chapter 1. Chapter 2 benefited from the expertise generously provided by Mary Gilchrist. I am indebted to Usha Balakrishnan who was also an early supporter and recruited R. Luke Evans and Sridhar Ramamoorti to review the initial version of the last chapter. I am grateful to Marianne Stratton who bailed me out at a point my secretarial skills foundered.

I cannot adequately express my gratitude to those who read all the chapters and offered cogent advice, including Holly Carver, Ronnye Wieland, Stanley Grant, Margaret Wolak, S. Derrickson Moore, and Jeffrey Murray. It is unlikely this effort would have progressed to publication without the in-depth understanding of the written material and the author's goals, as well the encouragement, of Jeffrey Murray. To all, I am most appreciative.

References

PREFACE

1. Deacon TW. Incomplete Nature: How Mind Emerged from Matter. W.W. Norton & Co., 2012, p. 143–81.

CHAPTER 1

1. Alt BL and Wells SK. Mountain Mafia: Organized Crime in the Rockies. Cold Tree Press, Nashville, Tennessee 2008.

2. Clagett OT and Geraci JE. A procedure for the management of postpneumonectomy empyema. J Thorac Carvdiovasc Surg 45:141, 1963.

3. Stafford EG, Clagett OT. Postpneumonectomy empyema: neomycin instillation and definitive closure. J Thorac Cardiovasc Surg 63:771, 1972.

4. Hodges A. Alan Turing: The Enigma. Vintage Books, London 2012.

5. Lester N. Stranger in Angel Town: A Pretty Eastern Schoolteacher in a Rough Rocky Mountain Town. Dodd, Meade & Company 1952.

6. Fennell JJ. They Called Them the Immortals: The Last of the Class. Lulu Press, Inc. 2017.

7. Lahr J. Tennessee Williams: Mad Pilgrimage of the Flesh. W. W. Norton & Company 2014.

8. Ludwig M. It's Perfectly Safe … : The RulisonMatter. Zafta Publishing, Downers Grove, IL. 2016, p. 161–5.

9. Dicker D. Shale Boom, Shale Bust: The Myth of Saudi America. Digital Edition 2015.

10. Wilczek F. A Beautiful Question: Finding Nature's Deep Design. Penguin Press 2015.

11. Thompson T. Hearts. Fawcett Publications, Greenwich, Conn. 1971.

12. Wade N. The Nobel Duel: Two Scientists' 21-Year Race To Win the World's Most Coveted Research Prize. Anchor Press/Doubleday, Garden City, NY 1981.

13. Carroll S. Brave Genius: A Scientist, a Philosopher, and Their Daring Adventures from the French Revolution to the Nobel Prize. Broadway Books 2014.

14. Jacob F and Monod J. Genetic regulatory mechanisms in the synthesis of proteins. J Mol Biol 3:318, 1961.

15. Doerner K. Pressure gradients in cells. J Theoret Biol 14:284, 1967.

16. Styron W. Darkness Visible: A Memoir of Madness. Random House, New York 1990.

17. Selye H. A syndrome produced by diverse nocuous agents. Nature 138:32, 1936.

18. Liebelt RA. Inbred mice fed only bee pollen. J of ApiProduct and ApiMedical Science 2:155, 2010.

19. Liebelt RA. A Story of My Bee Pollen Research in Mice and Humans. Windjammer Adventure Publishing, Chagrin Falls, OH 2015.

20. Pampallona S, Bollini P, Tibaldi G, Kupelnick B, Munizza C. Combined pharmacotherapy and psychological treatment for depression: a systematic review. Arch Gen Psy 61:714, 2004.

21. Solomon A. The Noonday Demon: An Atlas of Depression. Scribner 2001.

22. Stossel S. My Age of Anxiety: Fear, Hope, Dread, and the Search for Peace of Mind. Alfred A. Knopf, 2014.

23. Adams G, Williamson R, Harvey C, Murray R, and Hester R. Shallow habitat air diving with excursions between 5 and 250 FSWG: A review of four simulated dives. Underwater Physiology VI. (eds. Shilling CW and Beckett MW), 1978, p. 423–34.

24. Sontag S and Drew C. Blind man's Bluff: The Untold Story of American Submarine Espionage. Perennial 1998.

25. Subramanian S. A Dominant Character: The Radical Science and Restless Politics of J. B. S. Haldane. W. W. Norton & Co., 2020.

26. Ferris T. The Mind's Sky: Human Intelligence in a Cosmic Context. Bantam Books 1992.

27. Rippinger, Joel. The Benedictine Order in the United States: An Interpretive History. The Liturgical Press, Collegeville, MN., 1990.

28. Williamson TL and Crill WE. The effects of pentylenetetrazol on molluscan neurons. I. Intracellular recording and stimulation. Brain Research 116:217, 1976.

29. Williamson TL and Crill WE. The effects of pentylenetetrazol on molluscan neurons. II. Voltage clamp studies. Brain Research 116:231, 1976.

30. Motulsky AG, as told to King M-C. The great adventure of an American geneticist. Annual Review of Genomics and Human Genetics 17:1, 2016.

31. Hall JG. The clinic is my laboratory: Life as a clinical geneticist. Annual Review of Genomics and Human Genetics 18:1, 2017.

32. Hall JG, Sybert VP, Williamson RA, Fisher NL, Reed SD. Turner's syndrome. Western Journal of Medicine 137:32, 1982.

33. Karp LE. Genetic engineering: Threat or promise? Nelson-Hall 1976.

34. Karp LE. The view from the vue. Jonathan David Publishers 1977.

35. Oshinsky D. Bellevue: Three Centuries of Medicine and Mayhem at America's Most Storied Hospital. Doubleday 2016.

36. Karp LE. A cautionary tale for the discriminating reader. American Journal of Medical Genetics. 15:191, 1983.

37. Karp LE. David Smith: The pleasure of his company. American Journal of Medical Genetics. 8:263, 1981.

38. Hanson JW, Myrianthopoulos NC, Harvey MA, Smith DW. Risks to offspring of women treated with hydantoin anticonvulsants, with emphasis on the fetal hydantoin syndrome. Journal of Pediatrics 89:662, 1976.

39. Karp LE, Williamson RA, Moore DE, Shy KK, Plymate SR, Smith WD. The sperm penetration assay: A useful test in the evaluation of male fertility. Obstet and Gynecol 57:620, 1981.

40. Williamson RA, Koehler JK, Smith WD, Karp LE. Entry of immotile spermatozoa into hamster ova. Gamete Res 10:319, 1984.

41. Sulloway FJ. Freud, biologist of the mind: Beyond the psychoanalytic legend. Basic Books, Inc. 1979.

42. Andreasen NC. The Broken Brain: The Biological Revolution in Psychiatry. Harper & Row, New York 1984.

43. Foerstner A. James Van Allen: The first eight billion miles. University of Iowa Press 2007.

44. Gurnett DA, Kurth WS, Burlaga LF, Ness NF. In situ observations of interstellar plasma with Voyager I. Science 341:1489, 2013.

45. Bell J. The interstellar age: Inside the forty-year Voyager mission. Dutton 2015.

46. Williamson RA, Weiner CP, Yuh WTC, Abu-Yousef MM. Magnetic resonance imaging of anomalous fetuses. Obstet Gynecol 73:952, 1989.

47. Williamson RA, Varner, MW, Grant SS. A reduction in amniocentesis risks using a real-time/needle guide procedure. Obstet Gynecol 65:751, 1985.

48. Weiner CP, Wenstrom KD, Sipes SL, Williamson RA. Risk factors for cordocentesis and fetal intravascular transfusion. Am J Obstet Gynecol 165:1020, 1991.

49. Weiner CP, Williamson RA, ... Grant SS, Estle L. Management of fetal hemolytic disease by cordocentesis II. Outcome of treatment. Am J Obstet Gynecol 165:1302, 1991.

50. Wang F, Williamson RA, Mueller G, Thomas P, Davidson BL, McCray PB Jr. Ultrasound-guided gene transfer to hepatocytes in utero. Fetal Diagn and Ther 13:197, 1998.

51. Massaro G, Matlar CNZ, ... Waddington SN, Rahim AA. Fetal gene therapy for neurodegenerative diseases of infants. Nature Med 24:1317, 2018.

52. Williamson RA, Weiner CP, Ptil S, Benda J, Varner MW, Abu-Yousef MM. Abnormal pregnancy sonogram: Selective indication for fetal karyotype. Obstet Gynecol 69:15, 1987.

53. Clewell WH, Johnson ML, ... Henry GP, Shikes RH. A surgical approach to the treatment of fetal hydrocephalus. N Engl J Med 306:1320, 1982.

54. Williamson RA, Schauberger CW, Varner MW, Ashenbrenner CA. Heterogeneity of prenatal onset hydrocephalus: Management and counseling implications. Am J Med Genet 17:497, 1984.

55. Williamson RA. Fetal Surgery. In: Pitkin RM, Zlatnik FJ (Eds.): 1986 Yearbook of Obstetrics and Gynecology. Year Book Medical Publishers, Inc., Chicago, 1986, p. 219–48.

56. Williamson RA (Guest Ed.). Prenatal Diagnosis. In Clinical Obstetrics and Gynecology, Pitkin RM, Scott JM (Eds.): J. B. Lippincott Co., Philadelphia, 1988, p. 231–420.

57. Williamson RA, Murray JC. Molecular Analysis of Genetic Disorders. In: Pitkin RM, Scott JM (Eds.): Clinical Obstetrics and Gynecology. J. B. Lippincott Co., Philadelphia 31:270, 1988.

58. Ryan GL, Sparks AE, Sipe CS, Syrop CH, Dokras A, van Voorhis BJ. A mandatory single blastocyst transfer policy with educational campaign in a United States IVF program reduces multiple gestation rates without sacrificing pregnancy rates. Fertil Steril 88:354, 2007.

59. Braude P, Pickering S, Flinter F, Ogilvie CM Preimplantation genetic diagnosis. Nature Rev Genet 3:941, 2002.

60. Williamson RA, Elias S. Infertility and Pregnancy Loss. In: King RA, Rotter JL, Motulsky AG (Eds.): The Genetic Basis of Common Disease. McGraw Hill Book Co., 1992, 577–95.

61. Smithies A. Animal models of human genetic diseases. Trends in Gen 9:112, 1993.

62. Evans MJ, Kaufman MH. Establishment in culture of pluripotent cells from mouse embryos. Nature 292:154, 1981.

63. Smithies O, Gregg RG, Boggs SS, Koralewski MA, Kucherlapati RS. Insertion of DNA into the human chromosomal beta-globin locus by homologous recombination. Nature 317:230, 1985.

64. Shesely EG, Kim H-S, Shehee WR, Papayannopoulos T, Smithies O, Popovich BW. Correction of a human beta S-globin gene by gene targeting. Proc Natl Acad Sci USA 88:4294, 1991.

65. Williamson RA, Lee D, Hagaman J, Maeda N. Marked reduction of HDL cholesterol in mice genetically modified to lack apolipoprotein A-1. Proc Natl Acad Sci USA 89:7134, 1992.

66. Romero R. Giants in Obstetrics and Gynecology Series: A profile of Jennifer Niebyl, MD. Am J Obstet Gynecol 217:627, 2017.

67. Duclos F, Straub V, ...Williamson RA, Campbell KP. Progressive muscular dystrophy in α-sarcoglycan deficient mice. J Cell Biol 142:1461, 1998.

68. Sampaolesi M, Torrente Y, ... Bottinelli R, Cossu G. Cell therapy of α-sarcoglycan null dystrophic mice through intra-arterial delivery of mesangioblasts. Science 301:487, 2003.

69. Williamson RA, Henry MD, Daniels KJ, Hrstka RF, Lee JC, Sunada, Y, Ibraghimov-Beskrovnaya O, Campbell KP. Dystroglycan is essential for early embryonic development: Disruption of Reichert's membrane in Dag/-null mice. Hum Mol Genet 6:831, 1997.

70. Moore SA, Saito F, ...Williamson RA, Campbell KP. Deletion of brain dystroglycan recapitulates aspects of congenital muscular dystrophy. Nature 418:422, 2002.

71. Ackerman MJ, Clapham DE. Ion channels in basic science and clinical disease. New Engl J Med 336:1575, 1997.

72. Dickerson LW, Bonthius DJ, ...Williamson RA, Lamb FS. Altered GABAergic function accompanies hippocampal degeneration in mice lacking ClC-3 voltage-gated chloride channels. Brain Res 958:227, 2002.

73. Anderson MP, Gregory RJ, ... Smith AE, Welsh MJ. Demonstration that CFTR is a chloride channel by alteration of its anion selectivity. Science 253:202, 1991.

74. Snouwaert JN, Brigman KK, Latour AM, Malouf NN, Boucher RC, Smithies O, Koller BH. An animal model for cystic fibrosis made by gene targeting. Science 257:1083, 1992.

75. Trivedi BP. Breath from Salt. BenBella Books, Inc., 2020

76. Rogers CS, Stoltz DA, ...Prather RS, Welsh MJ. Disruption of the CFTR gene produced a model of cystic fibrosis in newborn pigs. Science 321:1837, 2008.

77. Cooney AL, Abou Alaiwa MH, ... Sinn PL, McCray PB Jr. Lentiviral-mediated phenotypic correction of cystic fibrosis pigs. J Clin Invest Insight 1:e88730, 2016.

78. McDonald FJ, Yang B, ...Welsh MJ, Williamson RA. Disruption of the β-subunit of the epithelial Na channel in mice: Hyperkalemia and neonatal death associated with a pseudohypoaldosteronism phenotype. Proc Natl Acad Sci USA 96:1727, 1999.

79. Ziemann AE, Allen JE, Welsh MJ, Wemmie JA. The amygdala is a chemosensor that detects carbon dioxide and acidosis to elicit fear behavior. Cell 139:1012, 2009.

80. Maren S. An acid-sensing channel sows fear and panic. Cell 139:867, 2009.

81. LeDoux J. Anxious: Using the Brain to Understand and Treat Fear and Anxiety. Viking 2015, p. 297.

82. Takahashi K, Yamanaka S. Induction of pluripotent stem cells from embryonic mice and adult fibroblast cultures by defined factors. Cell 126:663, 2006.

83. Takahashi K, Tanabe K, ...Tomoda K, Yamanaka S. Induction of pluripotent stem cells from adult human fibroblasts by defined factors. Cell 131:861, 2007.

84. Yu J, Vodyanik MA, ... Slukvin ll, Thomson JA. Induced pluripotent stem cell lines derived from human somatic cells. Science 318:1917, 2007.

85. Thomson JA, Itskovitz J, ... Marshall VS, Jones JM. Embryonic stem cell lines derived from human blastocysts. Science 282:1145, 1998.

86. Paşca SP. Assembling brain organoids. Science 363:126, 2019.

87. Turco MY, Gardner L, ... Henberger M, Burton GJ. Trophoblast organoids as a model for maternal-fetal interactions during human placentation. Nature 564:263, 2018.

88. Murray JC, Karp LE, Williamson RA, Cheng EY, Luthy DA. Rh isoimmunization related to amniocentesis. Am J Med Genet 16:527, 1983.

89. Kim YJ, Williamson RA, Murray JC, Andrews JL, Pietscher JJ, Peraud PJ, Merrill DC. Genetic susceptibility to preeclampsia: Roles of cytosine-to-thymine substitution at nucleotide 677 of the gene for methylenetetrahydrofolate reductase, 68-base pair insertion at nucleotide 844 of the gene for cystathionine-synthase, and Factor V Leiden mutation. Am J Obstet Gynecol 184:1211, 2001.

90. Kim YJ, Williamson RA, Chen K, Smith JL, Murray JC, Merrill DC. Lipoprotein lipase gene mutations and the genetic susceptibility of preeclampsia. Hypertension 38:992, 2001.

91. Murray JC, Buetow KH, ... Cohen D, Cann H: A comprehensive human linkage map with centimorgan density. Science 265:2049, 1994.

92. Williamson RA, Murray JC. Iowa's Role in the Genetics Revolution. In: As Far As the Eye Can See: The Promises and Perils of Research and Scholarship in the Twenty-first Century. Pradarelli, SJ (Ed.). University of Iowa Press 2019.

93. Bass GF, Throckmorton P, Taylor JDP, Hennessy JB, Shulman AR, Buchholz H-G. Cape Gelidonya: A Bronze Age Shipwreck. Transactions of the American Philosophical Society 57:1-177, 1967.

94. Pulak C. The Uluburun shipwreck: an overview. Inter J Naut Archeol 27:188, 1998.

95. Bass GF (Ed.). Beneath the Seven Seas: Adventures with the Institute of Nautical Archeology. Thames & Hudson 2005.

96. Bass GF. Archeology Beneath the Sea: My Fifty Years of Diving on Ancient Shipwrecks. Boyut Publishing 2013.

97. Fagan B. A Little History of Archeology. Yale University Press. 2018, p. 210–15.

98. Knauer K (Ed.) Great Scientists: The Geniuses, Eccentrics and Visionaries Who Transformed Our World. Time Books, New York, NY 2014.

99. Dubois L. Haiti: The After Shocks of History. Macmillan 2012.

100. Kidder T. Mountains Beyond Mountains: The Quest of Dr. Paul Farmer, a Man Who Would Cure the World. Random House 2003.

101. Rysavy MA, Bell EF, ... Brumbaugh JE, Higgins RD. Between-hospital variation in treatment and outcomes in extremely preterm infants. N Engl J Med 372:1801; 2015.

102. Younge N, Goldstein RF, ... Higgins RD, Cotten CM. Survival and neurodevelopmental outcomes among previable infants. N Engl J Med 376:617, 2017.

103. Kaluarachichi DC, Momany AM, ... Dagle JM, Rykkman KK, Murray JC. Polymorphisms in NR5A2 gene encoding liver receptor homolog-1 are associated with preterm birth. Ped Res 79:776, 2016.

104. Lander ES. The heroes of CRISPR. Cell 164:18, 2016.

105. Davies K. Editing Humanity: The CRISPR Revolution and the New Era of Genome Editing. Pegasus Books 2020.

106. Frangoul H, Altshuler D, ... Yen A, Corbacioglu S. CRISPR-Cas9 gene editing for sickle cell disease and beta-thalassemia. New Engl J Med 2020.

107. Boyden ES, Zhang F, Bambey E, Nagel G, Deisseroth K. Millisecond-timescale, genetically targeted optical control of neural activity. Nature Neurosc 8:1263, 2005.

108. Wietek J, Wiegert JS, ... Oertner TG, Hegemann P. Conversion of channelrhodopsin into a light-gated chloride channel. Science 344:409; 2014.

109. Tovote P, Fadok JP, Luthi A. Neuronal circuits for fear and anxiety. Nat Rev Neurosc 16:317, 2015.

110. Holstein J. The First Fifty Years at the Jackson Laboratory, 1929–1979. Bar Harbor: The Jackson Laboratory 1979.

111. Koller BH. Oliver Smithies (1925–2017). Cell 168:743, 2017.

112. Lawrence MG, Altenburg MK, ... Berg UB, Smithies O. Permeation of macromolecules into the renal glomerular basement membrane and capture by the tubules. Proc Natl Acad Sci 114:2958, 2017.

113. Carlson DN, Pulak C. George Fletcher Bass (1932–2021). Am J Archeol 125:1, 2021.

114. Wilson EO (Ed.). From So Simple a Beginning: The Four Great Books of Charles Darwin. W. W. Norton, New York 2005.

CHAPTER 2

1. Javaux EJ. Challenges in evidencing the earliest traces of life. Nature 572:451, 2019.

2. Knoll AH. Life on a Young Planet: The First Three Billion Years of Evolution on Earth. Princeton Univ Press 2003.

3. Fortey R. Life: A Natural History of the First Four Billion Years of Life on Earth. Alfred A. Knopf, Inc. 1997.

4. Zimmer C. Microcosm: E. coli and the New Science of Life. Pantheon Books 2008.

5. Pal RR, Baidya AK ... ... Ben-Yehuda S, Rosenshine I. Pathogenic E. coli extracts nutrients from infected host cells utilizing injectisome components. Cell 177:683, 2019.

6. Singla V, Reiter JF. The primary cilium as the cell's antenna: Signaling at a sensory organelle. Science 313:629, 2006.

7. Woese CR. On the evolution of cells. Proc Natl Acad Sci 99:8742, 2002.

8. Archibald J. One Plus One Equals One: Symbiosis and the Evolution of Complex Life. Oxford Univ Press 2014.

9. Lane N. Power, Sex, Suicide: Mitochondria and the Meaning of Life. Oxford Univ Press 2005.

10. Margulis L. Symbiotic Planet: A New Look. Basic Books, New York 1998.

11. Woese CR, Fox GE. Phylogenetic structure of the prokaryotic domain: the primary kingdoms. Proc Natl Acad Sci 74:5088, 1977.

12. Joyce GF. The antiquity of RNA-based evolution. Nature 418:214, 2002.

13. Yarus M. Life From an RNA World: The Ancestor Within. Harvard Univ Press 2010.

14. Martin WF, Sousa FL, Lane N. Energy at life's origin. Science 344:1092, 2014.

15. Lane N. The Vital Question: Why Is Life the Way It Is? Profile Books 2015.

16. Spang A, Saw JH.... ... .Guy L, Ettema TJG. Complex archaea that bridge the gap between prokaryotes and eukaryotes. Nature 521:173, 2015.

17. Williams TA, Foster PG, Cox CJ, Embley TM. An archael origin of eukaryotes supports only two primary domains of life. Nature 504:231, 2013.

18. Imachi H, Nobu MK ... ...Tamaki H, Taksi K. Isolation of an archaeon at the prokaryote-eukaryote interface. Nature 577:519, 2020.

19. Quammen D. The Tangled Tree: A Radical New History of Life. Simon & Schuster 2018.

20. Goldenfield N, Pace NR. Carl Woese (1928 – 2012). Science 339:661, 2013.

21. Gross M. Life on the Edge: Amazing Creatures Thriving in Extreme Environments. Plenum Press, New York 1996.

22. Falkowski PG, Fenchel T, DeLong EF. The microbial engines that drive earth's biogeochemical cycles. Science 320:1034, 2008.

23. Falkowski PG. Life's Engines: How Microbes Make Earth Habitable. Princeton Univ Press 2015.

24. Mitchell P. Coupling of phosphorylation to electron and hydrogen transfer by a chemiosmotic type of mechanism. Nature 191:144, 1961.

25. Pfeffer C, Larsen S.... ... ... Risgaard-Petersen N, Nielsen LP. Filamentous bacteria transport electrons over centimeter distances. Nature 49:218, 2012.

26. Camilli A, Bassler BL. Bacterial small-molecule signaling pathways. Science 311:1113, 2006.

27. Bassler BL, Losick R. Bacterially speaking. Cell 125:237, 2006.

28. Liu J, Prindle A, Humphries J. Garcia-Ojalvo J, Suel GM. Metabolic co-dependence gives rise to collective oscillations within biofilms. Nature 523:550, 2015.

29. Diggle SP, Griffin AS, Campbell, West SA. Cooperation and conflict in quorum-sending bacterial populations. Nature 450:411, 2007.

30. Moura-Aves P... ... ... Krause G, Kaufmann SHE. Host monitoring of quorum sensing during Pseudomonas aeruginosa infection. Science 366:1472, 2019.

31. Velcer GJ. Social strife in the microbial world. Trends in Microbiol 11:330, 2003.

32. Travisano M and Velicer GJ. Strategies of microbial cheater control. Trends in Microbiol 12:72, 2004.

33. Wilson EO. Sociobiology: The New Synthesis. Belknap Press of Harvard Univ Press 1975.

34. Parsek MR, Greenberg EP. Sociomicrobiology: the connections between quorum sensing and biofilms. Trends Microbiol 13:27, 2005.

35. Mashburn LM, Whiteley M. Membrane vesicles traffic signals and facilitate group activities in a prokaryote. Nature 437:422, 2005

36. Lyon P. The cognitive cell: bacterial behavior reconsidered. Front Microbiol 6:1, 2015.

37. Tagkopoulos I, Liu Y-C, Tavazoie S. Predictive behavior within microbial genetic networks. Science 320:1313, 2008.

38. Rust MJ, Golden SS, O'Shea EK. Light-driven changes in energy metabolism directly entrain the cyanobacterial circadian oscillator. Science 331:220, 2011.

39. Teng S-W, Mukherji S, Moffitt JR, de Buyl S, O'Shea EK. Robust circadian oscillations in growing cyanobacteria require transcriptional feedback. Science 340:737, 2013.

40. Blankenship RE. How cyanobacteria went green. Science 355:1372, 2017.

41. Aschoff J. Exogenous and endogenous components in circadian rhythms. Cold Spring Harbor Symp Quant Biol 25:11, 1960.

42. Pittendrigh CS. Temporal organization: Reflections of a Darwinian clock-watcher. Ann Rev Physiol 55:17, 1993.

43. Bell-Pederson D, Cassone VM ... ... Thomas TL, Zoran MJ. Circadian rhythms from multiple oscillators: Lessons from diverse organisms. Nature Rev Genet 6:544, 2005.

44. Bass J, Takahashi JS. Circadian integration of metabolism and energetics. Science 330:1349, 2010.

45. Man K, Loudon A, Chawla A. Immunity around the clock. Science 354:999, 2016.

46. Takahashi JS, Hong K-S, Ko CH, McDearmon EL. The genetics of mammalian circadian order and disorder: Implications for physiology and disease. Nature Rev Genet 9:765, 2008.

47. Li JZ, Bunney BG ... ... Akil H, Bunney WE. Circadian patterns of gene expression in the brain and disruption in major depressive disorder. Proc Natl Acad Sci 110:9950, 2013.

48. Panda S, Antoch MP ... ... Takahashi JS, Hogenesch JB. Coordinated transcription of key pathways in the mouse by the circadian clock. Cell 109:307, 2002.

49. Quin J, Raes LR ... ... Ehrlich SD, Wang J. A human gut microbial gene catalogue established by metagenomic sequencing. Nature 464:59, 2010.

50. Ley RE, Peterson DA, Gordon JI. Ecological and evolutionary forces shaping microbial diversity in the human intestine. Cell 124:837, 2006.

51. Dunn R. The Wild Life of Our Bodies: Predators, Parasites, and Partners That Shape Who We Are Today. HarperCollins Books 2015.

52. Gill SR, Pop M ... ... Fraser-Ligett CM, Nelson KE. Metagenomic analysis of the human distal gut microbiome. Science 312:1355, 2006.

53. Costello EK, Lauber CL, Hamady M, Fierer N, Gordon JI, Knight R. Bacterial community variation in human body habitats across space and time. Science 326:1694, 2009.

54. Sberro H, Fremin BJ ... ... Kyrpides NC, Bhatt AS. Large-scale analyses of human microbiomes reveal thousands of small, novel genes. Cell 178:1, 2019.

55. Rakoff-Nahoum S, Foster KR, Comstock LE. The evolution of cooperation within the gut microbiota. Nature 533:255, 2016.

56. Backhed F, Ding H, Wang T., Semenkovich CF, Gordon J I. The gut microbiota as an environmental factor that regulates fat storage. Proc Natl Acad Sci 101:15718, 2004

57. Barker D, Osmond C. Infant mortality, childhood nutrition, and ischaemic heart disease in England and Wales. Lancet 327:1077, 1986.

58. Li M, Falllin MD ... ... Zuckerman B, Wang X. The association of maternal obesity and diabetes with autism and other developmental disorders. Pediatr 137:e20152206, 2016.

59. Buffington SA, Di Prisco GV ... ... Petrosino JF, Costa-Mattioli M. Microbial reconstitution reverses maternal diet-induced social and synaptic deficits in offspring. Cell 165:1762, 2016.

60. Donaldson ZR, Young LJ. Oxytocin, vasopressin, and the neurogenetics of sociality. Science 322:900, 2008.

61. Sgritta M, Dooling SW ... ... Britton RA, Costa-Mattioli M. Mechanisms underlying microbial-mediated changes in social behavior in mouse models of autism spectrum disorder. Neuron 101:246, 2019.

62. Sherwin E, Borderstein SR, Quinn JL, Dinan TG, Cryan JF. Microbiota and the social brain. Science 366:587, 2019.

63. Vuong HE, Yano JM, Fung TC, Hsiao EY. The microbiome and host behavior. Annu Rev Neurosci 40:21, 2017.

64. Heijtz RD, Wang S ... ... Fossberg H, Pettersson S. Normal gut microbiota modulates brain development and behavior. Proc Natl Acad Sci 108:3047, 2011.

65. Valles-Colomer M, Falony ... ... Vieira-Silva S, Raes J. The neuroactive potential of the human gut microbiota in quality of life and depression. Nature Microbiol 4:623, 2019.

66. Gilbert JA, Blaser MJ ... ... Lynch SV, Knight R. Current understanding of the human microbiome. Nature Med 24:392, 2018.

67. Blaser MJ. Missing Microbes: How the Overuse of Antibiotics is Fueling Our Modern Plagues. Henry Holt and Company 2014.

68. Medzhitov R. Recognition of microorganisms and activation of the immune response. Nature 449:819, 2007.

69. Steinman R, Cohn ZA. Identification of a novel cell type in peripheral lymphoid organs of mice. I. Morphology, quantification, tissue distribution. J Exp Med 137:1142, 1973.

70. Lemaitre B, Nicolas NE, Michart L, Reichhart JM, Hoffman JA. The dorsoventral regularory gene cassette spatzle/Toll/cactus controls the potent antifungal response in Drosophila adults. Cell 86:973, 1996.

71. Poltorak A, Smirnova I ... ... Ricciardi-Castagnoli P, Beutler LB. Defective LPS signaling in C3H/10ScRr mice: Mutations in Tlr4 gene. Science 282:2085, 1998.

72. Hampton HG, Watson BN, Fineran PC. The arms race between bacteria and their phage foes. Nature 577:327, 2020.

73. Lee YK, Mazmanian SK. Has the microbiota played a critical role in the evolution of the adaptive immune system? Science 330:1768, 2010.

74. Gensollen T, Iyer SS, Kasper DL, Blumberg RS. How colonization by microbiota in early life shapes the immune system. Science 353:539, 2016.

75. Rakoff-Nahoum S, Pagline J, Eslami-Varzaneh F, Edberg S, Medzhitov R. Recognition of commensal micoroflora by Toll-like receptors is required for intestinal homeostasis. Cell 118:229, 2004.

76. Lathrop SK, Bloom SM ... ... Stappenbeck TS, Hsieh C-S. Peripheral education of the immune system by colonic commensal bacteria. Nature 478:250, 2011.

77. McFall-Ngai M. Care for the community. Nature 445:153, 2007.

78. Louveau A, Smirnov I ... ... Harris TH, Kipnis J. Structural and functional features of central nervous system lymphatic vessels. Nature 523:337, 2015.

79. Fung TC, Olson CA, Hsiao EY. Interactions between the microbiota, immune and nervous systems in health and disease. Nature Neurosc 20:145, 2017.

80. Thomas L. The Lives of a Cell: Notes of a Biology Watcher. The Viking Press 1974.

81. Marles-Wright, Grant T ... ... van Heel M, Lewis RJ. Molecular architecture of the "stressosome," a signal integration and transduction hub. Science 322:92, 2008.

CHAPTER 3

CHAPTER 3

1. Malakoff D. The rise of the mouse, biomedicine's model mammal. Science 288:248, 2000.

2. Tecott LH. The genes and brains of mice and men. Am J Psych 160:646, 2003.

3. Rader K. Making Mice: Standardizing Animals for American Biomedical Research, 1900–1955. Princeton Univ Press 2004.

4. Festing MEW, Fisher EMC. Mighty mice: Clarence Little's brainwave gave biomedical researchers their best friend. Nature 404:815, 2000.

5. McCray PB, Pewe L... ... ... Look DC, Perlman S. Lethal infection of K18hACE2 mice infected with severe acute respiratory syndrome coronavirus. J Virol 81:813, 2007.

6. Mouse Genome Sequencing Consortium: Initial sequencing and comparative analysis of the mouse genome. Nature 420:520, 2002.

7. International Human Genome Sequencing Consortium: Initial sequencing and analysis of the human genome. Nature 409:860, 2001.

8. Venter JC, Adams MD... ... ... Zandieh A, Zhu X. The sequence of the human genome. Science 291:1304, 2001.

9. King M-C, Wilson AC. Evolution at two levels in humans and chimpanzees. Science 188: 107, 1975.

10. Lein AS, Hawrylycz MJ... ... ... Zwingman TA, Jones AR. Genome-wide atlas of gene expression in the adult mouse brain. Nature 445:168, 2007.

11. Ng L, Bernard A... ... ... Jones AR, Hawrylycz M. An anatomic gene expression atlas of the adult mouse brain. Nat Neurosci 12:356, 2009.

12. Wang Q, Ding S-L... ... ... Harris JA, Ng l. The Allen mouse brain common coordinate framework: A 3D reference atlas. Cell 181:936, 2020.

13. Chung K, Wallace J... ... ... Gradinaru V, Deisseroth K. Structural and molecular interrogation of intact biological systems. Nature 497:332, 2013

14. Lee S-J, Lehar A... ... ... Liu Y, Germain-Lee EL. Targeting myostatin/activin A protects against skeletal muscle and bone loss during space flight. Proc Natl Acad Sci 117:23942, 2020.

15. Chen Z, Cheng K. Engleman JA, Wong K-K. A murine lung cancer coclinical trial identifies genetic modifiers of therapeutic response. Nature 483:613, 2012.

16. Milner B, Corkin S, Teuber H-L. Further analysis of the hippocampal amnesic syndrome. Neuropsychologia 10:1, 1968.

17. Dittrich L. Patient H.M. Memory, Madness, and Family Secrets. Penguin Random House 2017.

18. Kandel ER. In Search of Memory: The Emergence of a New Science of Mind. W.W. Norton & Co. 2006.

19. Bliss TVP, Lomo T. Long-lasting potentiation of synaptic transmission in the dentate area of anesthetized rabbit following stimulation of the perforant path. J Physiol (Lond.) 232:331, 1973.

20. Ho VM, Lee J-A, Martin KC. The cell biology of synaptic plasticity. Science 334:623, 2011

21. Kandel ER. The molecular biology of memory storage: a dialogue between genes and synapses. Science 294:1030, 2001.

22. Kandel ER, Spencer WA Cellular neurophysiological approaches to the study of learning. Physiol Rev 48:65, 1968.

23. Davis RL Physiology and biochemistry of Drosophila learning mutants. Physiol Rev 76:299, 1996.

24. Grant SGN, O'Dell TJ, Karl KA, Stein PL, Soriano P, Kandel ER. Impaired long-term potentiation, spatial learning, and hippocampal development in fyn mutant mice. Science 258:1903, 1992.

25. Silva AJ, Paylor P, Wehner JM, Tonegawa S. Impaired spatial learning in alpha-calcium-calmodulin kinase Il mutant mice. Science 257:206, 1992.

26. Tsien JZ, Chen DE ... ... Kandel ER, Tonegawa S. Subregion and cell-type restricted gene knockout in mouse brain. Cell 87:1317, 1966.

27. Tsien JZ, Huerta PT, Tonegawa S. The essential role of hippocampal CAI NMDA receptor-dependent synaptic plasticin in spatial memory. Cell 87:1327, 1996.

28. Kandel ER. Psychotherapy and the single synapse. N Engl J Med 301:1028, 1979.

29. Kandel ER. The Disordered Mind: What Unusual Brains Tell Us About Ourselves. Farrar, Straus, and Giroux 2018.

30. Valenstein ES. The War of the Soups and the Sparks. Columbia University Press 2005.

31. Buzsaki G. Rhythms of the Brain. Oxford University Press 2006.

32. Deisseroth K. Optogenetics: 10 years of microbial opsins in neuroscience. Nature Neurosci 18:1213, 2015.

33. Chalfie M, Tu Y, Euskirchen G, Ward WW, Prasher DC. Green fluorescent protein as a marker for gene expression. Science 263:802, 1994.

34. Heim R, Cubitt AB, Tsien RY. Improved green fluorescence. Nature 373:663, 1995.

35. Josselyn SA, Tonegawa S. Memory engrams: recalling the past and imagining the future. Science 367:39, 2020.

36. Zhou Y, Won J ... ... Poirazi P, Silva AJ. CREB regulated excitability and the allocation of memory to subsets of neurons in the amygdala. Nature Neurosc 12: 1438, 2009.

37. Han J-H, Kuishner SA ... ... Silva AJ, Josselyn SA. Neuronal competition and selection during memory formation. Science 316:457, 2007.

38. Wahlsten D. Mouse Behavioral Testing: How to Use Mice in Behavioral Neuroscience. Elsevier 2011.

39. Sah P, Westbrook RF. The circuit of fear. Nature 454:589, 2008.

40. Burgos-Robles A, Vidal-Gonzales l, Quirk GJ. Sustained conditioned responses in prelimbic prefrontal neurons are correlated with fear expression and extinction failure. J Neurosci 29:8474, 2009.

41. LeDoux J. The amygdala. Current Biol 17:R868, 2007.

42. Feinstein JS, Adolphs R, Damasio A, Tranel D. The human amygdala and the induction and experience of fear. Current Biol 21:34, 2011.

43. McGaugh JL. The amygdala modulates the consolidation of memories of emotionally arousing experiences. Annu Rev Neurosci 27:1, 2004.

44. Johansen JP, Hamanaka H ... ... Blair HT, LeDoux JE. Optical activation of lateral amygdala pyramidal cells instructs associative fear learning. Proc Natl Acad Sci 107:12692, 2010.

45. Tye KM, Prakash R ... ... Ramakrishnan C, Deisseroth K. Amygdala circuit mediating reversible and bidirectional control of anxiety. Nature 471:358, 2011

46. Ciocchi S, Henry C ... ... Muller C, Luthi A. Encoding of conditioned fear in central amygdala inhibitory circuits. Nature 468:277, 2010.

47. Etkin A, Prater KE, Schatzberg AF, Menon V, Greicius MD. Disrupted amygdalar subregion functional connectivity and evidence of a compensatory network in generalized anxiety disorder. Arch Gen Psych 66:1361, 2009.

48. Lebow MA, Chen A. Overshadowed by the amygdala: the bed nucleus of the stria terminalis emerges as key to psychiatric disorders. Molec Psych 21:450, 2016.

49. Kim S-Y, Abhikari A ... ... Tye KM, Deisseroth K. Diverging neural pathways assemble a behavioral state from separable features in anxiety. Nature 496:219, 2013.

50. Yehuda P. Post-traumatic stress disorder. New Engl J Med 346:108, 2002.

51. Lacagnino AF, Brockway ET ... ... Denny CH, Drew MR. Distinct hippocampal engrams control extinction and relapse of fear memory. Nat Neurosc 22:753, 2019.

52. Marshall M. Roots of mental illness. Nature 581:19, 2020.

53. Krishnan V, Nestler EJ. The molecular neurobiology of depression. Nature 455:894, 2008.

54. Disner SG, Beevers CG, Haigh EAP, Beck AT. Neural mechansims of the cognitive model of depression. Nature Rev Neurosci 12:467, 2011.

55. Stuber GD, Sparta DR ... ... Deisseroth K, Bonci A. Excitatory transmission from the amygdala to nucleus accumbens facilitates reward seeking. Nature 475:377, 2011

56. Tye KM, Mirzabekov JJ ... ... Witten IB, Deisseroth K. Dopamine neurons modulate neural encoding and expression of depression-related behavior. Nature 493:537, 2013.

57. Chaudhury D, Walsh JJ ... ... Nestler AJ, Han M-H. Rapid regulation of depression-related behaviors by control of midbrain dopamine neurons. Nature 493:532, 2013

58. Lammel S, Lim BK ... ... Tye KM, Deisseroth K. Input-specific control of reward and aversion in the ventral tegmental area. Nature 491:212, 2012.

59. LeGates TA, Kvarta MD ... ... Creed MC, Thompson SM. Reward behavior is regulated by the strength of hippocampus-nucleus accumbens synapses. Nature 564:258, 2018.

60. Ramirez S, Xu L, MacDonald CJ, Redondo RL, Tonegawa S. Activating positive memory engrams suppresses depression-like behavior. Nature 522:335, 2015.

61. Hirosaka O. The habenula: From stress evasion to value-based decision-making. Nature Rev Neurosci 11:503, 2010.

62. Li B, Piriz J ... ... Henn F, Malinow R. Synaptic potentiation onto habenula neurons in the learned helplessness model of depression. Nature 470:535, 2011.

63. Mayberg HS. Targeted electrode-based modulation of neural circuits for depression. J Clin Invest 119:717, 2009.

64. Tye KM, Deisseroth K. Optogenetic investigation of neural circuits underlying brain disease in animal models. Nature Rev Neurosci 13:251, 2012.

65. Berton O, Hahn C-G, Thase ME. Are we getting closer to valid translational models for major depression? Science 338:75, 2012.

66. Ziv L, Muto A ... ... Yamamoto KR, Baier H. An affective disorder in zebrafish with mutation of the glucocorticoid receptor. Molec Psych 18:681, 2013.

67. Warden MR, Selimbeyoglu A ... ... Frank LM, Deisseroth K. A prefrontal cortex-brainstem neuronal projection that controls response to behavioral challenge. Nature 492:428, 2012.

68. Notaras M, van der Buuse M. Neurobiology of DBNF in fear memory, sensitivity to stress, and stress-related disorders. Molec Psych 25:2251, 2020.

69. Berton O, McClung CA ... ... Self DW, Nestler EJ. Essential role of BDNF in the mesolimbic dopamine pathway in social defeat stress. Science 311:864, 2006

70. Krishnan V, Han M-H ... ... Gershenfeld HK, Nestler EJ. Molecular adaptations underlying susceptibility and resistance to social defeat in brain reward regions. Cell 131:391, 2007.

71. Liu, D, Diorio J ... ... Plotsky PM, Meaney MJ. Maternal care, hippocampal glucocorticoid receptors, and hypothalamic-pituitary-adrenal responses to stress. Science 277:1659, 1997.

72. Francis D, Diorio J, Liu D, Meaney MJ. Nongenomic transmission across generations of maternal behavior and stress responses in the rat. Science 286:1155, 1999

73. Weaver ICG, Cervoni N ... ... Szyf M, Meaney MJ. Epigenetic programming by maternal behavior. Nature Neurosci 7:847, 2004.

74. McGowan PO, Sasaki A ... ... Turecki G, Meaney MJ. Epigenetic regulation of the glucocorticoid receptor in human brain associates with child abuse. Nature Neurosci 12:742, 2009.

75. Agrawal AA. Phenotypic plasticity in the interactions and evolution of species. Science 294:321, 2001.

76. CONVERGE consortium. Sparse whole-genome sequencing identifies two loci for major depressive disorders. Nature 523:588, 2015.

77. Simonti CN, Vernot B ... ... Denny JC, Capra JA. The phenotypic legacy of admixture between modern humans and Neandertals. Science 351:737, 2016.

78. Kendler KS. What psychiatric genetics has taught us about the nature of psychiatric illness and what else is to learn. Molec Psych 18:1058, 2013

CHAPTER 4

1. Tovote P, Fadok JP, Luthi A. Neuronal circuits for fear and anxiety. Nature Rev Neurosci 16:317, 2015.

2. Shin LM, Liberzon I. The neurocircuitry of fear, stress, and anxiety disorders. Nueropsychopharm Rev 35:169, 2010.

3. LeDoux JE. The self: Clues from the brain. Ann NY Acad Sci 1001:295, 2003.

4. James W. What is an Emotion? Classics in the History of Psychology 2015. First published in Mind 9:188, 1884.

5. Adolphs R, Anderson DJ. The Neuroscience of Emotion: A New Synthesis. Princeton Univ Press 2018.

6. LeDoux J. The Deep History of Ourselves: The Four-Billion-Year Story of How We Got Conscious Brains. Viking 2019.

7. Damasio A. The Feeling of What Happens: Body and Emotion in the Making of Consciousness. Harcourt Brace & Co 1999.

8. Ekman P. Strong evidence for universals in facial expressions: A reply to Russell's mistaken critique. Psychological Bulletin 115:268, 1994.

9. Darwin C. The Expression of the Emotions in Man and Animals. Univ of Chicago Press 1872/1965.

10. Panskeep J. Affective Neuroscience: The Foundations of Human and Animal Emotions. New York: Oxford Univ Press 1998.

11. Janak PA, Tye KM. From circuits to behavior in the amygdala. Nature 517:284, 2015.

12. Nauta WJH, Karten HJ. A general profile of the vertebrate brain, with sidelights on the ancestry of the cerebral cortex. In Schmitt FO, ed. Neurosciences: Second Study Program. Rockefeller Univ Press 1970, p. 7–26.

13. Denton D. The Primordial Emotions: The Dawning of Consciousness. Oxford Univ Press 2005.

14. Craig AD. How do you feel? Interoception: The sense of the physiological condition of the body. Nature Rev Neurosci 3:655, 2002.

15. Dawkins R. The Extended Phenotype: The Long Reach of the Gene. Oxford Univ Press 1999.

16. Griffin DR. Animal Minds: Beyond Cognition to Consciousness. Univ of Chicago Press 2001.

17. Safina C. Beyond Words: What Animals Think and Feel. New York: Picador 2016.

18. Smith ML, Asada N, Malenka RC. Anterior cingulate inputs to nucleus accumbens control the social behavior of pain and analgesia. Science 371:153, 2021.

19. Burkett JP, Andari E, Johnson ZV, Curry DC, de Waal FBM, Young L J. Oxytocin-dependent consolation behavior in rodents. Science 351:375, 2016.

20. Anderson DJ, Adolphs R. A framework for studying emotions across species. Cell 157:187, 2014.

21. Venken KJ, Simpson JH, Bellen HJ. Genetic manipulation of genes and cells in the nervous system of the fruit fly. Neuron 72:202, 2011.

22. Anderson DJ. Circuit models linking internal states and social behavior in flies and mice. Nat Rev Neurosci 17:692, 2016.

23. Damasio A, Carvalho GB. The nature of feelings: evolutionary and neurobiological origins. Nature Rev Neurosci 14:143, 2013.

24. Shewmon DA, Holmes GL, Byrne PA. Consciousness in congenitally decorticate children: developmental vegetative state as self-fulfilling prophecy. Dev Med and Child Neurol 41:364, 1999.

25. Merker B. Consciousness without a cerebral cortex: A challenge for neuroscience and medicine. Behav and Brain Sci 30:63, 2007.

26. LeDoux JE. Rethinking the emotional brain. Neuron 73:653, 2012.

27. Hart D, Sussman RW. Man the Hunted: Primates, Predators, and Human Evolution. Westview Press 2005.

28. Barrett LF. How Emotions Are Made: The Secret Life of the Brain. Houghton Mifflin Harcourt 2017.

29. Damasio A. Self Comes to Mind: Constructing the Conscious Brain. Pantheon Books 2010.

30. Barrett LF. Are emotions natural kinds? Perspect Psychol Sci 1:28, 2006.

31. Phelps EA. Emotion and cognition: insights from studies of the human amygdala. Ann Rev Psychol 57:27, 2006.

32. Kim JJ, Diamond DM. The stressed hippocampus, synaptic plasticity and lost memories. Nature Rev Neurosci 3:453, 2002.

33. Arnsten AFT. Stress signalling pthways that impair prefrontal cortex structure and function. Nature Rev Neurosci 10:410, 2009.

34. Lau H, Rosenthal D. Empirical support for higher-order theories of conscious awareness. Trends Cogn Sci 15:365, 2011.

35. LeDoux JE, Brown R. A higher-order theory of emotional consciousness. Proc Natl Acad Sci 114: E2016, 2017.

36. Phelps EA, LeDoux JE. Contributions of the amygdala to emotion processing: from animal models to human behavior. Neuron 48:175, 2005.

37. LeDoux JE. In search of an emotional system in the brain: Leaping from fear to emotion and consciousness. In MS Gazzaniga (Ed.), The Cognitive Neurosciences. The MIT Press 1995, p. 1049–61.

38. Altman J, Das GD. Autoradiographic and histological evidence of postnatal hippocampal neurogenesis in rats. J Comp Neurol 124:319, 1965.

39. Spalding KL, Bergmann O... ... ... Drvid H, Frisen J. Dynamics of hippocampal neurogenesis in adult humans. Cell 153:1219, 2013.

40. Aimone JB, Li Y, Lee SW, Clemenson GD, Deng W, Gage FH. Regulation and function of adult neurogenesis: From genes to cognition. Physiol Rev 94:991, 2014.

41. Ming G, Song H. Adult neurogenesis in the mammalian brain: Significant answers and significant questions. Neuron 70:687, 2011.

42. Egeland M, Zunszain PA, Pariante CM. Molecular mechanisms in the regulation of adult neurogenesis during stress. Nat Rev Neurosci 16:189, 2015.

43. Hsieh J, Schneider JW. Neural stem cells, excited. Science 339:1534, 2013.

44. Hsieh J, Gage FH. Epigenetic control of neural stem cell fate. Curr Opin Genet Dev 14:461, 2004.

45. Gould E, Beylin A, Tanapat P, Reeves A, Shors TJ. Learning enhances adult neurogenesis in the hippocampal formation. Nat Neurosci 2:260, 1999.

46. Van Praag H, Kempermann G, Gage F. Neural consequences of environmental richness. Nat Rev Neurosci 1:191, 2000.

47. Van Praag H, Shubert T, Zhao C, Gage F. Exercise enhances learning and hippocampal neurogenesis. J Neurosci 25:8680, 2005.

48. Sahay A, Scobie KN... ... ... Dramovsky A, Hen R. Increasing adult hippocampal neurogenesis is sufficient to improve pattern separation. Nature 472:466, 2011.

49. Arruda-Carvalho M, Sakaguchi M, Akers KG, Josselyn SA, Frankland PW. Posttraining ablation of adult-generated neurons degrades previously acquired memories. J Neurosci 31:15113, 2011.

50. Shelie Y, Wany P, Gado M, Csermansky J, Vannier M. Hippocampal atrophy in recurrent major depression. Proc Natl Acad Sci 93:3908, 1996.

51. Jacobs BL, van Praag H, Gage FH. Adult brain neurogenesis and psychiatry: a novel theory of depression. Molec Psych 5:262, 2000.

52. Malberg JE, Eisch AJ, Nestler EJ, Duman RS. Chronic antidepressant treatment increases neurogenesis in adult rat hippocampus. J Neurosci 15:9104, 2000.

53. Santarelli L, Saxe M... ... ... Belzung C, Hen R. Requirement of hippocampal neurogenesis for the behavioral effects of antidepressants. Science 301:805, 2003.

54. Samuels BA, Hen R. Neurogenesis and affective disorders. Europ J Neurosci 33:1152, 2011.

55. Kendler KS, Karkowski LM, Prescott CA. Causal relationship between stressful life events and the onset of major depression. Am J Psych 156:837, 1999.

56. Snyder JS, Soumier A, Brewer M, Pickel J, Cameron HA. Adult hippocampal neurogenesis buffers stress responses and depressive behavior. Nature 476:458, 2011.

57. McEwen BS. Physiology and neurobiology of stress and adaptation: central role of the brain. Physiol Rev 87:873, 2007.

58. Anacker C, Luna VM ... ... Chen B, Hen R. Hippocampal neurogenesis confers stress resilience by inhibiting the ventral dentate gyrus. Nature 559:98, 2018.

59. Freund J, Brandmaier AM ... ... Lindenberger U, Kempermann G. Emergence of individuality in genetically identical mice. Science 340:756, 2013.

60. Wilson HV. On some phenomena of coalescence and regeneration in sponges. J Exp Zool 5:245, 1907.

61. Wagner DE, Wang IE, Reddien PW. Clonogenic neoblasts are pluripotent adult stem cells that underlie planarian regeneration. Science 332:811, 2011.

62. Paşca SP, Panagiotakos GP, Dolmetsch RE. Generating human neurons in vitro and using them to understand psychiatric disease. Ann Rev Neurosci 37:479, 2014.

63. Brennand KJ, Simone A ... ... Sebat J, Gage FH. Modelling schizophrenia using human induced pluripotent stem cells. Nature 473:221, 2011.

64. Wen Z, Nguyen HN ... ... Song H, Ming G-l. Synaptic dysregulation in a human iPS cell model of mental disorders. Nature 515:414, 2014.

65. Mirnics K, Middleton FA, Lewis DA, Levitt P. Analysis of complex brain disorders with gene expression microarrays: schizophrenia a disease of the synapse. Trends Neurosci 24:479, 2001.

66. Mertens J, Wang Q-W ... ... Gage FH, Yao J. Differential responses to lithium in hyperexcitable neurons from patients with bipolar disorder. Nature 527:95, 2015.

67. Kikuchi T, Morizane A ... ... Parmar M, Takahashi J. Human iPS cell-derived dopaminergic neurons function in a primate Parkinson's disease model. Nature 548:592, 2017.

68. Vadodaria KC, Ji Y ... ... Weinshilboum R, Gage FH. Altered serotonergic circuitry in SSRI-resistant major depressive disorder patient-derived neurons. Mol Psych 24:808, 2019.

69. Chen WV, Nwakeze CL ... ... Wu Q, Maniatis T. Pcdhac2 is required for axonal tiling and assembly of serotonergic circuitries in mice. Science 356:406, 2017.

70. Langer R, Vacanti JP. Tissue engineering. Science 260:920, 1993.

71. Brassard JA, Lutolf MP. Engineering stem cell self-organization to build better organoids. Cell Stem Cell 24:860, 2019.

72. Clevers H. Modeling development and disease with organoids. Cell 165:1586, 2016.

73. Grebenyuk S, Range A. Engineering organoid vascularization. Front Bioeng Biotechnol 7:39, 2019.

74. Wrighton PJ, Kiessling LL. Forces of change: mechanics underlying formation of 3D organ buds. Cell Stem Cell 16:453, 2015.

75. Takebe T, Enomura M ... ... Yoshikawa HY, Taniguchi H. Vascularized and complex organ buds derived from diverse tissues via mesenchymal cell-driver condensation. Cell Stem Cell 16:556, 2015.

76. Rowe RG, Daley GQ. Induced pluripotent stem cells in disease modelling and drug discovery. Nat Rev Genet 20:377, 2019.

77. Sato T, Clevers H. Growing self-organizing mini-guts from a single intestinal stem cell: mechanism and applications. Science 340:190, 2013.

78. Workman MJ, Mahe MM ... ... Holmrath MA, Wells JM. Engineered human pluripo-tent-stem-cell-derived intestinal tissues with a functional enteric system. Nat Med 23:49, 2017.

79. Saini A. Cystic fibrosis patients benefit from mini guts. Cell Stem Cell 19:425, 2016.

80. Paşca SP. The rise of three-dimensional human brain cultures. Nature 553:437, 2018.

81. Mariani J, Vaccarino FM. Breakthrough moments: Yoshiki Sasai's discoveries in the third dimension. Cell Stem Cell 24:837, 2019.

82. Suga H, Kadoshima T ... ... Oiso Y, Sasai Y. Self-formation of functional adenohy-pophysis in three-dimensional culture. Nature 480:57, 2011.

83. Sasai Y. Cytosystems dynamics in self-organization of tissue architecture. Nature 493:318, 2013.

84. Carmazine S, Deneubourg J-L, Franks NR, Sneyd J, Theraula G., Bonabeau E. In Self-Or-ganization in Biological systems. Princeton University Press 2001, p. 7–92.

85. Deacon TW. Incomplete Nature: How Mind Emerged From Matter. W.W. Norton & Co. 2012, p. 143–81.

86. Bhatia SN, Ingber DE. Microfluidic organs-on-a-chip. Nat Biotechnol 32:720, 2014.

87. Velasco S, Kedaigle AJ ... ... Levin JZ, Arlotta P. Individual brain organoids reproduc-ibly form cell diversity of the human cerebral cortex. Nature 570:523, 2019.

88. Mariana J, Coppola G ... ... Howe J, Vaccarino FM. FOXG1-dependent dysregulation of GABA/glutamate neuron differentiation in autism spectrum disorders. Cell 162:375, 2015.

89. Lancaster MA, Renner M ... ... Jackson AP, Knoblich JA. Cerebral organoids model human brain development and microcephaly. Nature 501:373, 2013.

90. Qian X, Nguyen HN, Song ... ... Song H, Ming G-I. Brain-region-specific organoids using mini-bioreactors for modeling ZIKA exposure. Cell 165:1238, 2016.

91. Sawada T, Chater TE ... ... Nikaido I, Kato T. Developmental excitation-inhibition imblalance underlying psychoses revealed by single-cell analyses of discordant twins-derived cerebral organoids. Molec Psych 25:2695, 2020.

92. Birey F, Anderson J ... ... Huguenard JR, Paşca SP. Assembly of functionally integrated human forebrain spheroids. Nature 545:54, 2017.

93. Brown EC, Clark DL, Hascel S, MacQueeng. Ramasubbu R. Thalamocortical connect-ing in major depressive disorder. J Affective Disord 217:125, 2017.

94. Xiang Y, Tanaka Y ... ... Weissman SM, Park I-H. hESC-derived thalamic organoids form reciprocal projections when fused with cortical organoids. Cell Stem Cell 24:487, 2019.

95. Hockmeyer D, Jaenisch R. Induced pluripotent stem cells meet genome editing. Cell Stem Cell 18:573, 2016.

96. Swank G, Koo B-K ... ... Beekman JM, Clevers H. Functional repair of CFTR by CRISPR/Cas9 in intestinal stem cell organoids of cystic fibrosis patients. Cell Stem Cell 13:653, 2013.

97. Trujillo CA, Rice ES ... ... Green RE Muotri AR. Reintroduction of the archaic variant of NOVA1 in cortical organoids alters neurodevelopment. Science 371:694, 2021.

98. Cannon W. The Wisdom of the Body. New York: W. W. Norton & Co., 1932.

99. Brannan S, Liotti M ... ... Denton D. Fox PT. Neuroimaging of cerebral activations and deactivations associated with hypercapnia and hunger for air. Proc Natl Acad Sci 98:2029, 2001.

100. Feinstein JS, Buzza C ... ... Tranel D, Wemmie JA. Fear and panic in humans with bilateral amygdala damage. Nat Neurosci 16:270, 2013.

101. Esquivel G, Schruers KR, Maddock RJ, Colasanti A, Griez EJ. Acids in the brain: a factor in panic? J Pshchopharm 24: 639, 2010.

102. Varming T. Proton-gated ion channels in cultured mouse cortical neurons. Neuropharm 38:1875, 1999.

103. Ziemann AE, Allen JE ... ... Welsh MJ, Wemie JA. The amygdala is a chemosensor that detects carbon dioxide and acidosis to elicit fear behavior. Cell 139:1012, 2009.

104. Maren S. An acid-sensing channel sows fear and panic. Cell 139:867, 2009.

105. Coryell MW, Wunsch AM ... ... Langbehn DR, Wemmie JA. Targeting ASIC1a reduces innate fear and alters neuronal activity in the fear circuit. Biol Psych 62:1140, 2007.

106. Wemmie J, Coryell M ... ... Sigmund C, Welsh MJ. Overexpression of acid-sensing ion channel 1a in transgenic mice increases fear-related behavior. Proc Natl Acad Sci 101:3621, 2004.

107. Coryell MW, Wunsch AM ... ... Langbehn DR, Wemmie JA. Acid-sensing channel-1a in the amygdala, a novel therapeutic target in depression-related behavior. J Neurosci 29:5381, 2009.

108. Wemmie JA, Chen J ... ... Freeman JH Jr, Welsh MJ. The acid-activated ion channel ASIC contributes to synaptic plasticity, learning, and memory. Neuron 34:463, 2002.

109. Zha X-m, Wemmie JA, Green SH, Welsh MJ. Acid-sensing ion channel 1a is a postsynaptic proton receptor that affects the density of dendritic spines. Proc Natl Acad Sci 103:16556, 2006.

110. Sloan SA, Darmanis S ... ... Barres BA, Paşca SP. Human astrocyte maturation captured in 3D cerebral cortical spheroids derived from pluripotent stem cells. Neuron 95:779, 2017.

111. Quadrato G, Nguyen T ... ... SA, Arlotta P. Cell diversity and network dynamics in photosensitive human brain organoids. Science 545:48, 2017.

112. Trujillo CA, Gao R ... ... Voytek B, Muotri AR. Complex oscillatory waves emerging from cortical organoids model early human brain network development. Cell Stem Cell 25:558, 2019.

113. Farahany NA, Greely HT. The ethics of experimenting with human brain tissue. Nature 556:429, 2018.

114. Hyun I. Engineering ethics and self-organizing models of human development: opportunities and challenges. Cell Stem Cell 21:718, 2017.

115. Reardon S. Can lab-grown brains become conscious? Nature 586:658, 2020.

116. Jack AI, Shallice T. Introspective physicalism as an approach to the science of consciousness. Cognition 79:161, 2001.

117. Perkel JM. Single-cell analysis enters the multiomics age. Nature 595;614, 2021.

CHAPTER 5

1. Diagnostic and Statistical Manual of Mental Disorders. Fifth Ed. American Psychiatric Publishing 2013, p. 302–6.

2. Hunter ECM, Sierra M, David AS. The epidemiology of depersonalization and derealization: A systematic review. Soc Psychiatry Epidemiol 39:9, 2004.

3. Sierra M, Medford N, Wyatt G, David A. Depersonalization disorder and anxiety: A special relationship? Psychiatry Res 197:123, 2012.

4. Radovic F, Radovic S. Feelings of unreality: A conceptual and phenomenological analysis of the language of depersonalization. Philosophy, Psychiatry, & Psychology 9:271, 2002.

5. Rescher N. The Riddle of Existence. Univ Press of Amer 1984, p. 2.

6. Vesuna J, Kauvar IV............ Parvizi J, Deisseroth K. Deep Posteromedial cortical rhythm in dissociation. Science 586:87, 2020.

7. Larson D, Dunkley J............ Wollack E, Wright EL. Seven-year Wilkinson microwave anisotropy probe (WMAP) observations: Power Spectra and WMAP-derived parameters. Astrophys J Supp 192:1, 2011.

8. Hubble E. A spiral nebula as a star system, Messier 31. Astrophys J 69:103, 1929.

9. Fixen DJ, Hinshaw G, Bennett CL, Mather JC. The spectrum of the cosmic microwave background anisotropy from the combined COBE FIRAS and DMR observations. Astrophys J 486:623, 1997.

10. Smoot GF, Bennett CL............ WeissR, Wilkinson DT. Structure in the COBE DMR first year maps. Astrophys J 396: L1, 1992.

11. Perlmutter S, Aldering G, Goldhaber G, Knop RA, Nugent P, Castro PG. Measurements of and from 42 high-redshift supernovae. Astrophys J 517:565, 1999.

12. Reiss AG, Filippenko AV............ Suntzeff NB, Tonry J. Observational evidence from supernovae for an accelerating universe and a cosmological constant. Astronom J 116:1009, 1998.

13. Kirschner RP. The Extravagant Universe: Exploding Stars, Dark Energy and the Accelerating Cosmos. Princeton Univ Press 2004.

14. Mack K. The End of Everything (Astrophysically Speaking). Scribner 2020.

15. Higgs PW. Spontaneous symmetry breakdown without massless bosons. Phys Rev 145:1156, 1996.

16. Aad G, Abajyan T............ Zutshi V, Zwalinski L. Observation of a new particle in the search for the Standard Model Higgs boson with the atlas detector at the LHC. Physics Letters B 716:1, 2012.

17. Chatrchyan S, Khachatryan V............ Swanson J, Wenman D. Observations of a new boson at a mass of 125 GeV with the CMS experiment at the LHC. Physics Letters B 716:30, 2012.

18. Carroll S. The Particle at the End of the Universe: How the Hunt for the Higgs Boson Leads Us To the Edge of a New World. Dutton 2012.

19. Livio M. Why symmetry matters. Nature 490:472, 2012.

20. Wilczek F. A Beautiful Question: Finding Nature's Deep Design. Penguin Press 2015.

21. Johnson JA. Populating the periodic table: Nucleosynthesis of the elements. Science 363:474, 2019.

22. Yin J, Cao Y, Li Y-H............ Wang J-Y, Pan J-W. Satellite-based entanglement distribution over 1200 kilometers. Science 356:1140, 2017.

23. Feynman R. The Character of Physical Law. MIT Press 1967, p. 129.

24. Lederman L. The God particle et al. Nature 448:310, 2007.

25. Zurek W. Quantum Darwinism. Nature Physics 5:181, 2009.

26. Krauss L. A Universe From Nothing: Why there is Something Rather Than Nothing. Free Press 2012.

27. Wilczek F. The cosmic asymmetry between matter and antimatter. Scientific Amer 243:82, 1980.

28. Gefter A. Trespassing On Einstein's Lawn: A Father, a Daughter, the Meaning of Nothing and the Beginning of Everything. Bantam Books 2014.

29. Wheeler JA. At Home in the Universe. Amer Institute of Physics Press 1994, p. 292–4.

30. Rovelli C. Relational quantum mechanics. Internat J of Theoretical Physics 35:1637, 1996.

31. Rovelli C. Reality Is Not What It Seems: The Journey to Quantum Gravity. Riverhead Books (trans. from Italian). 2017.

32. Haldane JBS. Possible Worlds. 1927, p. 298.

33. Barrett LF. How Emotions Are Made: The Secret Life of the Brain. Houghton Mifflin Harcourt 2017.

34. LeDoux J. The Deep History of Ourselves: The Four-Billion-Year Story of How We Got Conscious Brains. Viking 2019.

35. Schacter DL, Addis DR. The cognitive neuroscience of constructive memory: remembering the past and imagining the future. Phil Trans R Soc B 362:773, 2007.

36. Schacter DL. Searching for Memory: The Brain, the Mind, and the Past. Basic Books 1996.

37. Barrow JD. The Infinite Book: A Short Guide to the Boundless, Timeless, and Endless. Vintage Books 2005.

38. Pascal B. Penses, Trans A. Krailsheimer, Penguin, London 1966.

39. Friedman M, ed. Martin Buber's Life and Work: The Early Years 1878–1923. E.P. Dutton, NY 1981.

40. Crick F, Koch C. A framework for consciousness. Nat Neurosci 6:119, 2003.

41. Eichenbaum H. On the integration of space, time, and memory. Neuron 95:1007, 2017.

42. Moser EI, Kropff E, Moser M-B. Place cells, grid cells, and the brain's spatial representation system. Annu Rev Neurosci 31:69, 2008.

43. MacDonald CJ, Lepage KQ, Eden UT, Eichenbaum H. Hippocampal "time cells" bridge the gap in memory for discontinuous events. Neuron 71:737, 2011.

44. Tsao A, Sugar J... ... ... Moser M-B, Moser EI. Integrating time from experience in the lateral entorhinal cortex. Nature 561:57, 2018.

45. Allison HE. Kant's Transcendental Idealism. Yale Univ Press 2004.

46. Wills TJ, Cacucci F, Burgess N, O'Keefe J. Development of the hippocampal cognitive map in preweanling rats. Science 328:1573, 2010.

47. Langston RF, Ainge JA... ... ... Moser E, Moser M-B. Development of the spatial representation system in the rat. Science 328:1576, 2010.

48. Holt J. Why Does the World Exist? An Existential Detective Story. W.W. Norton & Co. 2012.

49. Penrose R. Shadows of the Mind. Oxford Press 1994.

50. Al-Khalili J, McFadden J. Life On the Edge: The Coming Age of Quantum Biology. Bantam Press 2014.

51. Lane N. The Vital Question: Why Is Life the Way It Is? Profile Books 2015.

52. Panitchayangkoon G, Voronine DV... ... ... Mukamel S, Engel GS. Direct evidence of quantum transport in photosynthetic light-harvesting complexes. Proc Natl Acad Sci 108:20908, 2011.

53. Mouritsen H. Long-distance navigation and magnetoreception in migratory animals. Nature 558:50, 2018.

54. Xu J, Jarocha LE, Zollitsch T... ... ... Mouritsen H, Hare PJ. Magnetic sensitivity of cryotpchrome 4 from a migratory songbird. Nature 594:535, 2021.

55. Cook ND. The neuron-level phenomena underlying cognition and consciousness: synaptic activity and the action potential. Neurosci 153:556, 2008.

56. Denton D. The Primordial Emotions: The Dawning of Consciousness. Oxford Univ Press 2005, p. 235.

57. Koch C, Massimini M, Boly M, Tononi G. Neural correlates of consciousness: progress and problems. Nat Rev Neurosci 17:307, 2016.

58. Chalmers DJ. Facing up to the problem of consciousness. J Consc Studies 2:200, 1995.

59. Goff P. Galileo's Error: Foundations for a New Science of Consciousness. Pantheon Books 2019.

60. Eddington AS. The Nature of the Physical World. London: Macmillan 1928.

61. Russell B. The Analysis of Matter. London: Kegan Paul 1927.

62. Schrodinger E. What Is Life? The Physical Aspect of the Living Cell. Cambridge Univ Press 1944.

63. Davies P. A quantum recipe for life. Nature 437:819, 2005.

64. Gurnett DA, Kurth WS, Burlaga LF, Ness NF. In situ observations of interstellar plasma with Voyager 1. Science 341:1489, 2013.

65. Bell J. The Interstellar Age: Inside the Forty-Year Voyager Mission. Dutton 2015 p. 254.

Index

Albuquerque, NM, 65, 66
ACC. *See* cortex: anterior cingulate (ACC)
acid sensing, 96, 193
acidosis, 193
action potential, 125
acute respiratory syndrome 2.
    See SARS-CoV-2
Adams, George, 56–58
addiction, 157
adenosine triphosphate (ATP), 119
Adolphs, Ralph, 166, 168, 170–71, 172
air (compressed), 58–59
air embolism, 59
air hunger, 167, 168, 192–93
air pressure, 41, 62–63
Allen, Paul, 140
Allen Institute, 140
alphaproterobacteria, 117
Alvin (submersible), 102
amino acids, 115, 147, 190–91
Ammerman, Mary, 15
amniocentesis, 70, 75, 83
amygdala, 96, 150–52, 156, 167, 174, 189
    acid sensing in, 96, 193
    basolateral, 151, 169
    central nucleus, 151
    emotions and, 150–51, 152, 167, 193
    extended (*see* BNST)
Anderson, David, 166, 168, 170–71, 172
Andreasen, Nancy, 79
anhedonia, 156, 157
animals
    consciousness and, 168–69, 171, 174, 176
    learning and, 137–61
    memory and, 29, 127, 143–44
    migration of, 214
antibiotic resistance, 114, 129

antibodies, 130, 145
antidepressants, 156, 179, 184
antigens, 130, 131, 132
antimatter, 208
Anvil Points, CO, 14–15
anxiety, 42, 107, 142, 149, 154, 155
    acid sensing and, 96, 193
    microbiome and, 127
    MRIs and, 153
anxiogenesis, 150
anxiolysis, 150, 153
Anxious (LeDoux), 96, 193
Aplysia californica, 143–44, 149
apolipoprotein A-1, 89
archaea, 115, 116–18, 131
archaebacteria. *See* archaea
archeology
    dating techniques, 177
    underwater, 60–61, 65, 95, 100, 109
ASD. *See* autism spectrum disorder (ASD)
ASIC1a gene. *See* genes: ASIC1a
asymmetries, 208, 209
ATP. *See* adenosine triphosphate (ATP)
ATP synthase, 120
autism spectrum disorder (ASD), 126, 127,
    188
autobiography, ix, x
autoimmunity, 130, 133

Bacillus subtilis, 122, 134
bacteria, 32, 115, 116–17, 123, 131, 167
    cheating, 122
    cognition and, 123
    communication/cooperation between,
    118–23
    competition and, 122
    CRISPR/Cas and, 105–6

evolutionary relationships, 115–16
fingerprinting, 115, 116
internal 24-hour clock, 123
luminous, 121
polymerase chain reaction and, 106
symbiotic relationships, 121
bacterial speech bubbles, 123
Ballard, Robert, 102–3
Barker hypothesis. *See* fetal programming
Barnard, Christiaan, 38
barophiles, 116
Barrett, Lisa Feldman
    her theory of constructed emotion,
        173–74, 210
Bass, Ann, 59, 61, 101
Bass, George, 59–62, 100–102, 109
Baylor College of Medicine, Houston,
    37–39, 138
BDNF, 160–61, 177
Beautiful Question, A (Wilczek), 205
bed nucleus of the stria terminalis (BNST).
    See BNST
behavioral despair, 156
behaviors
    comforting, 169
    defensive, 151, 167
    emotions and, 166, 169
    maternal, 161
    social, 126–27
Bell, Ed, 104–5
Bell, Jim
    Interstellar Age, 219
Bell, Marie, 5–6, 7, 11, 15, 53
Bell, Raymond, 5–6, 7, 11, 15
Bellevue Hospital, New York, 75
Ben Taub Hospital, Houston, 53, 75
Benedictine Monastery (Our Lady of
    Guadalupe Abbey), Pecos, 67–68
Berberich, Stanton, 81
Beutler, Bruce, 131
Big Bang, 202–3
Bill (partner of Tom Williamson), 2, 68
bioenergetics, 119
biofilm, 121–22
biogeochemical cycles, 118–19
biology
    emergence, x, 187

molecular, 99, 100
    quantum mechanics and, 213, 214–15, 218
bioluminescence, 121–22, 148
bipolar disorder, 183–84
black holes, 213
Blaser, Martin, 128–29
blastocysts, 88–89
BNST, 153
Bodrum, Turkey, 60–61
Bodrum Museum of Underwater
    Archeology, Turkey, 61
Boebert, Lauren, 28
Book Cliffs, Rifle, CO, 13
bosons, 204, 205
brain, x, 43, 46, 140, 194, 195, 215–16
    acid-based status and panic disorder, 193,
        197–98
    anxiety and, 150–54
    construction of emotions and, 173–74
    deep stimulation of, 159
    development of, 149, 195
    dopamine reward pathway, 157
    fear and, 150–54, 175, 176
    forebrain, 197
    fusion of regions, 189
    interaction with environment, 212
    mice, 140–41, 180–81
    microbiome and, 127–28, 133–34
    mid-, 172
    neural pathways, 107, 127, 153–54, 157
    organoids of, 98, 176, 191, 195–98
    panic attacks and, 52, 191–92
    plasticity, 176, 181
    receipt of interoception signals, 168
    reward processes in, 157
    temporal lobe, 189
    wave frequencies synchronization, 174
    See also amygdala; bed nucleus of
        the stria terminalis (BNST); cortex;
        habenula; hippocampus; insula
brain-derived neurotrophic factor (BDNF).
    See BDNF
bromodeoxyuridine (BrdU), 178
Buber, Martin, 211
Buresh, Chris, 103

Campbell, Kevin, 94, 97
cancer
    cervical, 104
    ovarian, 2–3, 69–70, 72, 80
    See also fibrosarcoma
Cannon, Walter, 191
Cape Gelidonya project, Turkey, 100–101
Capecchi, Mario, 87, 93, 144
carbohydrates, 118
Carbon-14, 177
Carlson, Deborah, 109
Carroll, Sean
    Particle at the End of the Universe, The,
    205, 206–7
Castle, William, 138
Catcher in the Rye (Salinger), 26
Cedars-Sinai Medicine Center,
    Los Angeles, 71
cells, 134, 148, 181
    alteration of, 88–89
    B, 130
    clocks within, 123–24
    dedifferentiation of, 97, 114
    dendritic, 131
    differentiation of, 181
    "face," 212
    germ, 182
    "grid," 212
    host, 122
    immune, 195
    ion channels and, 95, 96, 193–94, 215
    mesenchymal, 185, 186, 195
    "mirror," 212
    neural crest, 186
    place, 212
    plasticity of, 96, 97, 143, 149, 152, 156
    presence of nuclei or not, 115
    pyramidal, 142, 145, 152
    red blood (RBCs), 83
    retinal, 195
    T, 130–31, 133
    "time," 212
    vascular, 195
    vertebrate, 113
    See also engrams; neurogenesis; neurons;
    stem cells
Cepheid variables, 202

Cerise, Coston, 25
Cesarean sections, 129
CF. *See* cystic fibrosis (CF)
Chalfie, Martin, 148
Chalmers, David, 216
Charpentier, Emmanuella, 106
chemical messaging, 125–26
chloride, 186
chlorophyll, 118
chloroplast, 118
cholesterol, 89
Christo, 31
cilia, 113
circadian rhythms, 123–24, 214
cirrhosis, 1–2
Clagett, O. F., 7–8
Clagett, O. T. (Jim), 7
Clagett procedure, 8
CLARITY, 141
Clifford, Betty
    Rifle Vignettes, 13, 31
clocks (internal), 123–24
clonal expansion, 130
cloning, 96
CNS. *See* nervous system: central
CO_2, 168, 192–93
coevolution, 127–28, 132
cognition, 123, 173, 175, 180
Collett, Robert (Bob), 16
Collins, Francis, 99–100
Colorado State University, Fort Collins, 33
communication, 118–23
    microbiome and, 127
Community Health Initiative, 103
compasses, 215
conditional targeting, 144
conditioned place preference, 158
conditioning
    Pavlovian/classical, 143, 144, 149–50, 156, 170
    context fear, 150
    freeze response from, 149
confidence, 90–91
consciousness, ix–x, 111, 165–69, 174, 175, 176,
    192, 194–98, 199, 210, 211–12, 213, 215–20
    animals and, 168–69, 174
    binding problem of, 210–11
    dualism versus materialism approaches, 210,

electromagnetism, 204, 206, 214–15
electrons, 119–20, 214–15
electrophoresis, 108
elements, 206
elevated maze plus test, 150
embryoid bodies, 88, 181–82
embryology, 181, 185
embryos, 106, 107
emergence, x, 187
emotional primitives, 171
emotions, 163, 165–98
    amygdala and, 150–51, 152, 167, 193
    biological bases of, x, 150–51, 170, 175–76
    cognitive awareness and, 173
    construction of, 173–76, 210
    dysregulation of, x, 163, 165, 174
    feelings versus, 166, 170, 174
    primary, 167
    primordial, 167, 192
    secondary/social, 167
    See also anxiety; fear
empathy, 9–10, 169
endosymbiont, 117
endosymbiosis, 114, 117
energy (chemical), 114, 117, 118, 119–20
Englert, François, 205
engrams, 148, 154, 158, 159
entanglement, 206, 215, 218
environment, ix–x
    extreme, 116
    genetics and, 42, 74, 76, 111, 161–62, 178
    neural interactions, 212
    navigation within, 212
enzymes, 214
epigenetics, 161–62, 178
    maternal behavior and, 161
epinephrine, 151
ES cells: *See* stem cells: embryonic (ES)
Escherischia coli. See *E. coli*
eukaryotes, 115, 116, 117, 148
Evans, Martin, 88, 93
evolution, 109–10, 113–15, 139, 155, 167, 173
    human, 113, 117, 139, 162
    mice, 139
experiences, 216
explosions (thermonuclear), 203–4
extinction training, 154

Extravagant Universe, The (Kirschner), 203
extremophiles, 116
Exxon Mobil, 31

Falkowski, Paul, 118
Farmer, Paul, 103
fate determination, 177
fear, 167, 174, 175, 176, 196
    case of S. M., 151, 192–93
    existential, 175
    processing of/memories of, 96, 107, 149–54, 175, 192
    resilience to, 96, 193
feelings, 166–67, 170, 174
Fennell, John, 17
fetal anemia, 83
Fetal Diagnosis and Therapy Clinic, Iowa City, 99
Fetal Hydantoin Syndrome, 76
fetal programming, 126
fetoscopy, 77–78
fetuses
    diaphragmatic hernia, 84
    neural tube defects, 84
    surgery, 54, 77, 84–86
    treatment of, 83–85
Feynman, Richard, 206
fibroblasts, 96–97, 98, 183
fibrosarcoma, 69–70
flagella, 112–13, 120
flying, 62, 88, 89–90
fMRI, 156, 159
free association, 44, 45
freeze response, 149, 152, 160
Freud, Sigmund, 45
    Interpretation of Dreams, 78
From So Simple a Beginning (Wilson), 110
Frost, Honor, 100
fruit flies, 131

GABA, 147, 188, 189, 195
Gable, Dan, 80
Gage, Fred, 177, 182–83, 184
gamma-aminobutyric acid (GABA). *See* GABA
Garfield County Fair and Rodeo, Rifle, CO, 20–21, 22

disease, 89
transplants, 38
hepatitis B, 2, 17
Higgs, Peter, 204
Higgs boson, 204, 205
Higgs field, 205
higher order theory (HOT), 174–75
Hi-Ho Café, Georgetown, CO, 19
Hilgers, Robert, 69, 104
hippocampus, 95, 142–43, 147, 150, 152, 156,
   157, 161–62, 174, 178–79, 180, 189, 212
   dentate gyrus, 177, 180
   dorsal sector, 180
   mnemonic functions of, 174
   ventral sector, 180
Hoffman, Jules, 131
holobiont, 125
Holt, Jim
   Why Does the World Exist?, 213
homeostasis, 191–92
hominids (extinct), 162, 190–91
homologous recombination, 88, 89, 106–7,
   108
homosexuality, 8–9, 17, 37
Honduras, 104
hormones, 152
   glucocorticoid, 152, 160, 178, 180
   stress, 51, 160
HOT. *See* higher order theory (HOT)
Howard Hughes Medical Institute, 94
Hoyle, Fred, 202
Hubble, Edwin, 202
Hubble Space Telescope, 203
hubris, 64, 78
Hughes, Howard, 94
"Human and Mammalian Genetics
   and Genomics: The McKusick Short
   Course," 108
humans
   commonalities with mice, 87, 89, 94, 139,
      141, 149
   evolution, 113, 117, 139
   genome, 99, 139–40
   genome editing, 107
   microbiome and, 125–29, 133
Hurricane Sandy, 138
hydranencephaly, 172

hydrocephalus, 84–85
hygiene hypothesis, 128
hyperarousal, 154
hyperbaric chambers
   mice experiments, 41–42, 46, 47
hypopituitarism, 187
hypothalamus, 124, 126, 180
hypoxia, 93

Illing, Waldemar, 100, 101
immune system, 128, 129–34
   adaptive/acquired, 129, 130, 131–32, 133,
      145
   communication between innate and
      adaptive/acquired, 130
   innate, 129–30, 131
In Search of Memory (Kandel), 143
in vitro fertilization (IVF), 86
INA. *See* Institute of Nautical Archeology,
   Bodrum
induced pluripotent stem cells (IPSCs). *See*
   stem cells: induced pluripotent (IPSCs)
infants, 104–5
infections, 130, 131
Infinity, 16, 211
inflammation, 132
inflammatory bowel disease, 133
information replication, 218
injectisome, 113
insects, 170
inside/outside dichotomy, 208
Institute of Nautical Archeology, Bodrum,
   61–62, 100, 101, 109
insula, 168
International Fetal Medicine and Surgery
   Society (IFMSS), 84
International Space Station, 141
interneurons, 147, 153, 189
interoception, 168, 171
Interpretation of Dreams (Freud), 78
Interstellar Age (Bell), 219
invertebrates, 133, 143
ion channels, 95, 201, 215
   ASIC1a, 96, 193–94
Iowa City, IA, 80
IPSCs. *See* stem cells: induced pluripotent
   (IPSCs)

Maeda, Nobuyo, 87–88, 89, 108, 181
magnetoreception, 214
mantle shelf, 144
Margulis, Lynn, 114
Martha (girlfriend of Roger Williamson), 36
Martin, Robert, 35–36, 39, 44
mass, 205
materialism, 210, 215–16, 218
Maternal Serum Pregnancy Screening
    Program, IA, 99
Mather, John, 202, 204
matter, 208
McCray, Paul, 139
McKusick, Victor, 72, 73, 108
Meaney, Michael, 161
medical genetics, 70–79, 86
    counseling, 50, 70, 74, 75, 76
    ethics and, 75–76, 82, 100, 107
    obstetrics and, 70–71
medical school
    stress of, 6, 42–45, 49, 51–52
medicine
    hyperbaric, 54, 60
    personalized, 185, 186
meditation, 209–10
Meeker Massacre, 14
meiosis, 88
memory and memories, 19, 137, 142–46,
    147–48, 178–79, 194, 210–11, 212
    animal, 23, 127, 143–44
    consolidation (long-term), 144
    emotion-laden, 152, 158
    episodic, 212
    explicit, 142, 152
    formation (short-term), 144
    implicit, 142, 143–44
    neurogenesis and, 178–79
    optogenetics and, 148–55
    PTSD and, 154
    stored (see engrams)
"Memory engrams" (Josselyn and
    Tonegawa), 148
Mendeleev, Dmitri, 206
Mendels' laws, 138
Messer, Robert, 65, 70
metabolism, 124
metabolites, 127, 128, 195

metacognition, 173, 175
methane, 115–16
methanogens, 115–16
methylation, 161–62
mice, 163
    anhedonia in, 156, 157, 180
    antidepressants and, 156, 184
    anxiety in, 128, 149–50, 153, 178
    behavioral despair, 156, 157, 158, 180
    brain, 140–41, 153, 154, 169
    breeding, 137–38, 139
    bullied, 156
    coat colors, 137, 138
    colonies, 108
    commonalities with humans, 87, 89, 94,
        139, 141, 149
    depression in, 155–62, 179–80
    diet, 126–27
    dissociative behavior, 201
    distribution of, 138
    elevated maze plus test, 150
    empathy and, 169
    exercise and, 178
    fear and, 96, 193
    fear learning and memory, 107, 149–50,
        153, 169
    forced swim test, 155–56, 157, 180
    "freezing" as a response, 149
    genes/genetics, 138, 140, 141, 178
    germ-free, 128, 132
    hyperbaric chambers experiments with,
        41–42, 46, 47, 57, 87
    inbred strains, 138
    knocked out (KO), 88–89, 94, 95–96, 106,
        141, 145
    learned helplessness of, 156, 157
    learning and, 178
    memory of, 96, 107, 144, 149, 158 178–79
    microbiomes, 126–28
    modelling with, 105, 126–27, 137, 138–41
    motor activity, 128
    nerves, 141
    neural maps of, 145
    neural pathways experiments with, 107,
        153–54
    neurogenesis in, 178–81
    open field test, 150

neurotransmission, 147, 184
neurotransmitters, 43, 125, 134, 157, 183, 189
Niebyl, Jennifer, 87, 91
nitrogen narcosis, 58
Nobel Prize in Chemistry, 106, 120, 148
Nobel Prize in Physics, 202, 203, 205, 213
Nobel Prize in Physiology or Medicine, 93, 123, 130–31, 143, 145, 213
norepinephrine, 43, 151, 157
Nothingness, 16, 200, 207–8, 209, 210, 211
nuclear forces, 206
nucleus, 115, 119
nucleus accumbens (NAc). *See* NAc

oil shale, 13, 14–15, 30–31, 56
O'Keefe, John, 212
olfaction, 177
ontology, 199, 200, 218
open field test, 150
Opitz, John, 76
opsins, 107, 146, 147, 158, 160
optogenetics, 107, 146, 147–55, 156, 157–58, 169, 201
organ buds, 185–86
organoids, 181, 185–91
  brain, 98, 176, 186, 188, 191, 195–98
  consciousness and, 195–98
  culturing, 185
  fusion of, 189–90
  intestinal, 186, 190
  thalamic, 189–90
  3D, 185, 186
  trophoblast, 98
organ-on-a-chip, 187
oscillators, 124
ovaries, 182
oxidation, 119
oxygen, 117, 118, 119, 123
oxytocin, 126–27, 170

panic and panic attacks, 23–24, 42, 52, 191–92, 196–97
panpsychism, 216–18
Panskeep, Jaak, 167, 168, 171
Parkinson's disease, 183, 184
Particle at the End of the Universe, The (Carroll), 205, 206–7

particle physics, 206–7, 208, 213–14
  Standard Model (SM), 204
Partners in Health, 103
Pascal, Blaise, 211
pathogen-associated molecular patterns (PAMPs), 129–30, 131, 132–33
pathways
  dopamine reward, 157–58, 184
  hippocampus-amygdala-NAc, 158
  hypothalamus-pituitary-adrenal, 134, 151–52, 159
  molecular, 160
  neural, 107, 127, 153–54, 157, 159, 170–71
  serotonin, 184
  signal transduction, 123
  stress, 161, 180
  VTA-medial prefrontal cortex, 158
  VTA-NAc, 158
Patil, Irene, 82
Patil, Shiva, 81–82
pattern separation, 178
Paul D. Wellstone Muscular Dystrophy Cooperative Center, Iowa City, 97
Pavlov, Ivan, 149–50
Peercy, David, 25, 26, 32
Penrose, Roger, 213, 215
  Shadows of the Mind, 213
periodic table, 206
Perlman, Stanley, 139
Perlmutter, Saul, 203
pH, 116
pharmacogenetics, 73
phase transitions, 191, 205, 207
phenotypes, 141, 161, 162, 168
photons, 204–5
photosynthesis, 118, 177, 214
phylogenetics, 115
physics, 34
  See also particle physics
pigs, 96
Pitkin, Roy, 86, 87
pituitary gland, 186–87
placenta, 98
planaria, 181
plants, 118
plasma wave instrument, 80
plasticity, 96, 97, 127, 149, 152, 156, 158, 176

University of Iowa Medical School, Iowa City, 79–80
 chromosome laboratory, 81
 Fetal Diagnosis and Therapy Clinic, 99
 Fetal Diagnosis and Treatment Unit, 81, 98
 Gene Targeting Core Facility, 91, 94, 95–96, 97
 Maternal Fetal Medicine (MFM) division, 98
 Paul D. Wellstone Muscular Dystrophy Cooperative Center, 97
 Reproductive Endocrine division, 86
University of New Mexico School of Medicine, Albuquerque, 63
University of North Carolina Medical School, Chapel Hill, 86–89, 109
University of Washington School of Medicine, Seattle, 71–72
unreality, 45–46, 199, 210, 218–19
uranium, 31
Urbach Wiethe syndrome, 151
Utes, 14

vaccines, 138–39
vagus nerve, 127
Valley Curtain (artwork), Rifle, CO (Christo), 31
Van Allen, James, 80
Van Allen radiation belts, 80
Van Voorhis, Bradley, 86
vanadium, 31
Vasa (ship), 95
Vasa Museum, Stockholm, 95
vascularization, 185, 186
ventral tegmental area (VTA). *See* VTA
vents (undersea hydrothermal), 116–17
vertebrates, 133
Vibrio fischeri, 121
viruses, 105–6, 131–32
 corona, 137–39
 as delivery systems for genes, 84, 194
 Zika, 188
vision, 107, 146, 211
 binding problem of, 210
Vital Question, The (Lane), 119–20
Vogel, Friedrich, 73

voles, 169–70
Voyager I mission, 80, 219
Voyager II mission, 80, 219
VTA, 157–58

Weiner, Carl, 83, 98
Weir, Robert, 100
Wellstone, Paul D., 97
Welsh, Michael, 94, 95–96
Wemmie, John, 96
What is an Emotion? (James), 166
What is Life? (Schrödinger), 218
Wheeler, John Archibald, 207, 208
Why Does the World Exist? (Holt), 213
Wilczek, Frank, 34, 208
 Beautiful Question, A, 205
Williams, Tennesse, 79
 Glass Menagerie, The, 26–27
Williamson, Arthur, 4–5
Williamson, Georgeanne, 4, 5, 18
Williamson, Marilyn. *See* Latham, Marilyn (Williamson)
Williamson, Mary Ann, 104
Williamson, Roger A.,
 childhood, 6–20
 high school, 21–32
 undergraduate school, 33–36
 medical school and internship, 37–53
 Navy, 54–64
 residency, 65–71
 fellowship, 72–80
 medical school faculty and retirement, 81–110

Williamson, Tim, 2, 7, 9, 10, 13, 15, 17, 24–25, 34, 51–54, 65, 104
Williamson, Tom, 1–2, 4–9, 5, 10, 11–12, 18–19, 24, 28, 33, 37, 44, 50–51, 54, 66-68
Wilson, E. O., 122
 From So Simple a Beginning, 110
Wilson, H. V., 181
Winokur, George, 79
Woese, Carl, 114–16, 118
 fingerprinting of bacteria, 115, 116
Women's Global Cancer Alliance, 104
Wood, Michael, 63–64

About the Author

After graduating from Baylor College of Medicine in Houston, Texas, with MD and MS degrees, Roger Williamson completed a pediatric internship, followed by a stint in the Navy performing diving and hyperbaric medicine research. A residency in obstetrics and gynecology was followed by a fellowship in medical genetics. He has been on the faculty at the University of Iowa Carver College of Medicine where he is currently an emeritus professor. In addition to clinical work largely focused on ultrasound, fetal diagnosis and treatment, and genetic counseling, he established a research program directed toward gene targeting, the inactivation of specific genes in mice to determine gene function and to produce mouse models of human genetic disease. These and other activities have fostered a broad interest in science and its implications for our lives.

Made in the USA
Middletown, DE
19 July 2023

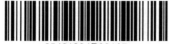

35421384R00165